A History of the Royal Hospital Chelsea 1682–2017

They Shall Not Grow Old, As Those That Are Left Grow Old:
Age Shall Not Weary Them, Nor The Years Condemn.
At The Going Down Of The Sun And In The Morning
We Will Remember Them.

A History of the Royal Hospital Chelsea 1682–2017

The Warriors' Repose

Stephen Wynn and Tanya Wynn

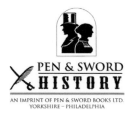

PEN & SWORD
HISTORY

AN IMPRINT OF PEN & SWORD BOOKS LTD.
YORKSHIRE – PHILADELPHIA

First published in Great Britain in 2019 by
Pen & Sword History
An imprint of
Pen & Sword Books Limited
Yorkshire - Philadelphia

Hardback ISBN 978 1 52672 0 177
Paperback ISBN 978 1 52675 1 447

A CIP catalogue record for this book is available from the British Library

Typeset in Ehrhardt by
Aura Technology and Software Services, India

Printed and bound in the UK
by TJ International Ltd, Padstow, Cornwall

Pen & Sword Books Limited incorporates the imprints of Atlas,
Archaeology, Aviation, Discovery, Family History, Fiction, History,
Maritime, Military, Military Classics, Politics, Select, Transport, True Crime,
Air World, Frontline Publishing, Leo Cooper, Remember When, Seaforth
Publishing,
The Praetorian Press, Wharncliffe Local History, Wharncliffe Transport,
Wharncliffe True Crime and White Owl.

For a complete list of Pen & Sword titles please contact
PEN & SWORD BOOKS LIMITED
47 Church Street, Barnsley, South Yorkshire S70 2AS, United Kingdom
E-mail: enquiries@pen-and-sword.co.uk
Website: www.pen-and-sword.co.uk

Or
PEN AND SWORD BOOKS
1950 Lawrence Rd, Havertown, PA 19083, USA
E-mail: Uspen-and-sword@casematepublishers.com
Website: www.penandswordbooks.com

Contents

Introduction

This book came about because of a visit that my wife and I made to the Royal Hospital Chelsea to speak with one of the in-pensioners in April 2017. It was my first experience of having the privilege of being at this great institution; as for my wife, it was a place she had visited a few times over the years, including the Chelsea Flower Show as a child. I found it an awe-inspiring place, a mixture of historic architecture, gardens and grounds.

We arrived in plenty of time for our meeting with one of the hospital's well-known residents on a lovely, sunny Spring morning, and as we were early we went for a coffee, sitting amongst many of the pensioners, who were talking to each other without an apparent care in the world.

As our visit was coming to an end, we bade our host goodbye and meandered through the hospital's cemetery on our way out. As we stood reading the names on the headstones of some of the great and good who had lived and died here over the centuries, my wife turned to me and smiled before uttering those immortal words, 'we should write a book about this place'. The rest, as they say, is history.

The extensive history connected to the Royal Hospital makes it such an enjoyable subject to write about. There is a wealth of available information, it is more a case of what to leave out rather than what to include.

Writing about the Royal Hospital Chelsea means having to include so many people from different eras of history and so many levels of the social spectrum to tell the whole story of this historic and iconic military, medical facility. The journey begins with such luminaries as Henry VIII, before moving on to Charles II. Then it was the turn of Christopher Wren and a look at the hospital's numerous governors, many of whom had the added credentials of having had illustrious military careers, one of them a recipient of the highest British military award for valour, the Victoria Cross.

The First and Second World Wars saw the Royal Hospital a victim of German air raids, which resulted in many casualties, both dead and injured.

There have been numerous ex-soldiers who have been residents of the hospital over the centuries, both men and women clad in the famous scarlet coloured tunic. Don't dare be lax and refer to it as being red, at least not within earshot of one of the pensioners, or you will be politely corrected.

No book on the Royal Hospital Chelsea would be complete without including the story of Margaret Thatcher's connection with this home for veterans, especially as the Infirmary has her name emblazoned above the doorway and her ashes were buried in the garden immediately outside at 11.30am on Saturday, 28 September 2013.

To finish the book by being as up to date as possible, we have taken a brief look at some of those who were either residents at the hospital, or who worked there in some capacity during the period of writing throughout 2017.

Hopefully, by the time you have finished this book you will have found it an enjoyable and interesting read, one that has given you an insight and a flavour of the Royal Hospital Chelsea and the numerous people who across the centuries have become part of its history and are forever woven into the very fabric of what this great institution is all about.

This book is dedicated to the memory of all those who have been residents at the hospital, as well as those who have worked there or been connected to it in some way.

Tanya and Stephen would like to thank all those who have helped them with the compilation of this book, with a special thanks to in-pensioner Paul Whittick for his invaluable assistance and friendship.

Chapter 1

The Beginning

The Royal Hospital Chelsea was the brainchild of King Charles II who founded it in 1682 as a retreat for injured veterans of his armies who had fought wars on his behalf. It is still going strong to this day as the home of the world-famous Chelsea Pensioners, where retired soldiers of the British Army are offered care and comradeship in their twilight years in recognition of their loyal service to the nation.

Prior to the building of the Royal Hospital, there was already a building, albeit an unfinished one, on the site. It was intended to be Chelsea College for theologians, the idea for which had come from King James I in 1609.

To understand the need for such a hospital, one has to look back to the Dissolution of the Monasteries that took place between 1536 and 1541 during the reign of King Henry VIII. At the time Henry was married to Catherine of Aragon, the first of his six wives, who was his queen from June 1509 until May 1533, but because she could not provide him with a son and heir, he tired of her. She had previously been married to Henry's elder brother, Arthur, the Prince of Wales and heir apparent. They had married in 1501 when she was just 16 years of age and Arthur was only 15, a marriage that by today's standards would not legally be permitted.

After their marriage they lived together at Ludlow Castle in Shropshire, but just five months later, and without warning, Arthur died. History records that his ailment was the 'Sweating Sickness', thought to have been brought over by mercenaries in the pay of Henry VII when he sailed to England to wrest the crown from Richard III at the Battle of Bosworth. There were a number of epidemics of it, beginning in 1485, the year of the battle, some in England and others across Europe.

Catherine would later claim that her marriage to Arthur had not been consummated, and by the time Henry attempted to use the fact that he believed it had been so as to obtain a divorce from Catherine, it was too late to disprove.

In 1525 Henry VIII became infatuated with Anne Boleyn, the daughter of Thomas Boleyn, 1st Earl of Wiltshire. But there were three problems: Henry was by now the King of England; he was a married man and Anne was not prepared just to become his mistress, like her sister Mary. Henry now had to find a way to be able to marry Anne. The most obvious option was to have Catherine murdered, but if he did and was found out, he would have had any even bigger problem on his hands, as Catherine's father was Ferdinand II, King of Spain. It would have undoubtedly have led to a bloody war between the two states.

Although Henry and Catherine had a daughter, Mary, who in July 1553, became Queen Mary 1 of England and Ireland, at the time when she was Henry's heir presumptive there was no established precedent for a woman to become queen in her own right. Henry decided that the only way that he could marry Anne Boleyn, was to have his marriage to Catherine annulled. He appealed to Pope Clement VII in Rome, but he refused Henry's request.

Henry's response was unforeseen. He simply made himself, and all subsequent English monarchs, the Supreme Head of the Church of England; prior to this the position had been held by the Pope in Rome. The first Act of Supremacy which allowed Henry to act as he did, was passed into law by Parliament on 3 November 1534. It also required an oath of loyalty from subjects recognising his marriage to Anne Boleyn. So it was that the Archbishop of Canterbury, Thomas Cranmer, granted Henry his divorce, a matter in which he had no real say. This decision led to England breaking away from the Roman Catholic Church.

Part of the way in which the Church amassed its fortunes was to charge people for religious services, such as marriages, baptisms and burials, as well as what were known as 'indulgences', pardons for sins committed, condemned by the German Protestant reformer Martin Luther. Belief in God in the sixteenth century was absolute and to speak out or go against the teachings of the Church meant risking the wrath of God, or so people believed, and to do that meant the possibility of not being allowed into heaven, which was simply unthinkable.

The Catholic Church was extremely rich; it had money, land and property and plenty of all three. This moment in time coincided with King Henry needing large sums of money to finance his military campaigns throughout the 1540s, provide a regular income for the Crown, and also to pay for his personal expensive tastes. The monies were literally there for the taking and that is exactly what he did.

The country was awash with religious houses in the mid-1530s; there were some 900 of them. These included 260 monasteries for monks, 300 churches or properties for canons, 142 convents for nuns and 183 friaries. This accounted for a total of 12,000 men and women, which meant that at the time one adult male in every fifty of the population was in some kind of religious order.

As a result of the Suppression of Religious Houses Act of 1539, wealthier monasteries were closed, along with the hospitals, leper houses and almshouses which had developed around them and which for centuries past had cared for the old, sick and infirm. A number of these individuals were retired soldiers, who were too old to fight or had been wounded in battle, and could not work and provide for themselves and their families. So it was that a decision made by one king in the early 1530s, resulted in a future king in the shape of Charles II founding the Royal Hospital in the late 1600s, specifically for veterans who had served their king and country when called upon to do so.

Charles II, or the 'Merry Monarch' as he is also referred to, was born on 29 May 1630 at St James's Palace in London. When he was 19 years of age, his father, King Charles I, was executed at Whitehall on 30 January 1649, having lost the English Civil War to the armies of the English and Scottish Parliaments. He surrendered to Scottish forces who then handed him over to the English Parliament, but he refused their demands for a constitutional monarchy and was imprisoned. He escaped, albeit briefly, in November 1647 and on his recapture, he was imprisoned on the Isle of Wight. There he forged an alliance with Scotland, but Oliver Cromwell, having taken control of England, had Charles I tried for high treason against England by using his power and position as king, to pursue his own personal interests, rather than those of the country. The case was prosecuted by the Solicitor General, John Cook. Part of the charge against him was that he waged war against Parliament and the people whom they represented, a war in which an estimated 300,000 people were killed.

His trial began on 20 January 1649 at Westminster Hall, London. In the end he was found guilty of high treason and sentenced to death. The day of his execution arrived, 30 January 1649, a cold winter's morning. He had been held at St James's Palace and was walked under guard the short distance to the Palace of Whitehall where his execution would take place. To ensure that nobody thought he was showing fear as he walked calmly to his death in the cold air of a winter's morning, he had worn two shirts to prevent him from shivering. At 2pm that day his head was severed from his body by one clean stroke. The following day his head was sewn back on to his body which was then embalmed and placed in a lead coffin.

The monarchy was abolished and a republic was declared and given the name of the Commonwealth of England.

Charles II was proclaimed King of Scotland on 5 February 1649 by the Scottish Parliament, but his position was short lived, for soon he was engaged in a civil war with Oliver Cromwell and his roundheads, the climax being at the Battle of Worcester on 3 September 1651. Cromwell's Parliamentarian New Model Army, a disciplined force of full-time professional soldiers, some 28,000 in number, were up against only 16,000 Royalist troops, who were

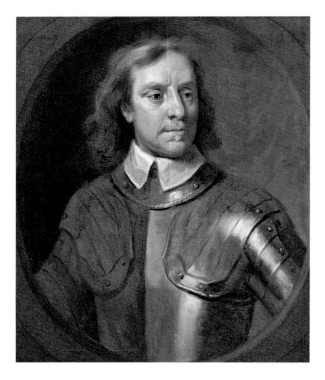

Figure 1: Oliver Cromwell.

mainly Scottish, and under the overall command of Charles II. They were well and truly routed, which resulted in Charles fleeing abroad, which he managed to do in part due to the help of Jane Lane, who, on marrying Sir Clement Fisher on 8 December 1663, became Lady Fisher. Sir Clement and Jane were married by the Archbishop of Canterbury.

She, in fact, played a heroic part in King Charles II's escape after his defeat at the Battle of Worcester, which in the circumstances was no mean feat. There was an immediate reward of £1,000 offered for the king's capture, which was a staggering amount of money at the time, and it is very likely that anybody found aiding and abetting his escape, would have been executed with him. Cromwell's soldiers were scouring the countryside, hoping that it would be they who would capture the wanted king. A big disadvantage for Charles was his height. In an age when the vast majority of men were not particularly tall, maybe 5ft 8in to 5ft 10in, at the most, he was some 6ft 2in tall and had a darker complexion than most other Englishmen.

When Charles II escaped after the Battle of Worcester, he did so with several others, two of whom were Lord Derby and Lieutenant General Henry Wilmot, 1st Earl of Rochester. Wilmot made his way alone to the home of Colonel John Lane, who was an officer in King Charles's Royalist Army, hoping that he would be in a position to help the king escape. Whilst with Colonel Lane, Wilmot learned that his sister, Jane Lane, a Catholic, had obtained a permit from the military authorities for herself and a servant to travel to Bristol, where she was due to visit a relative, Ellen Norton, who was with child and soon to give birth. The need for a permit was because it was illegal for Catholics to travel more than five miles from their homes without a pass from the sheriff of the county where they lived.

On learning of Jane's intended visit to Bristol, Wilmot came up with the idea for King Charles to go with her, pretending to be her servant and, once in Bristol, make good his escape by boat across the English Channel to France. It was a good idea, but one fraught with danger for Jane Lane and meant certain death if Charles's true identity should be discovered.

Charles arrived at John Lane's home at Bentley Hall, at Walsall in the early hours of 10 September 1651, and was appraised by Wilmot of the audacious plan of escape. He was dressed in common clothes and took the name William Jackson. In addition to Jane Lane and the king, disguised as her servant, there were her sister, Withy Petre, her husband, John Petre and Henry Lascelles, a Royalist officer, whilst Lord Wilmot, although part of the group, rode some distance ahead to act as a look out.

The journey was not without its problems. At one stage the horse that Jane Lane and the king were riding, shed a shoe, which needed repairing, and so the king had to take it to the local blacksmith to have the horse re-shod. Thankfully, no suspicions were raised. At Wootton Wawen on 10 September, the party had to calmly ride through a group of Cromwell's soldiers, as they approached the local Inn.

Their destination, Abbots Leigh, the home of Jane Lane's friend, Ellen Norton and her husband George, was reached on the evening of 12 September. Despite the fact that Jane Lane remained with them for three days, the Nortons were not aware that the King of England was in their midst, believing instead that the man who had accompanied Jane Lane, was nothing more than the servant he purported to be. Charles and Wilmot did not waste their time whilst Jane Lane was visiting her heavily pregnant friend; they went to the port of Bristol looking for a ship that was due to be sailing for France, but to no avail.

With the situation looking grave, destiny intervened and made it a whole lot worst, when Mrs Ellen Norton, unexpectedly, had a miscarriage. The Nortons were hoping that in the circumstances Jane would be able to stay with them whilst Ellen recovered, but the king had to move on if Wilmot was to help make good His Majesty's escape via another port, and for that they needed the presence of Jane Lane. To this end a letter had to be fabricated, purportedly from her brother, requesting that she urgently returned home to Bentley Hall.

On 16 September 1651 Charles II, still a lowly servant, left the Norton's home with Jane Lane and Henry Lascelles, supposedly on their way back to Bentley Hall. Instead they made their way to Trent in Dorset, via Castle Cary, arriving there the following day, and made their way to the home of another Royalist officer, Colonel Francis Wyndham, who lived at Trent House. Whilst Charles and Wilmot remained as guests of Colonel Wyndham, Jane Lane and Henry Lascelles, returned to Bentley Hall.

Word somehow reached the authorities that Jane had helped the king escape and now she was in danger. As soon as she was made aware of the precarious situation that she found herself in, she left Bentley Hall, and made her way to Yarmouth on foot, pretending to be nothing more than a common wench, making good her escape and finally arriving in Paris in December 1651. She was welcomed at Charles's court in exile, by both him and his wife, Queen Henrietta Maria.

Some time in the early part of 1652, Jane moved on to Holland, where she became a lady in waiting to Charles's sister, Princess Mary, where she remained until Charles had returned to England and been restored as king on the death of Oliver Cromwell.

Charles spent nine years living in exile in France, in what was then known as the Spanish Netherlands and the Dutch Republic. In his absence, Cromwell was the virtual dictator of England, Scotland and Ireland. It was only after his death on 3 September 1658, of septicaemia following a urinary infection, that Charles was able to consider returning to Britain, which he finally did on 29 May 1660, receiving a rousing reception on his arrival in London. At his coronation on 23 April 1661, he was crowned King of England, Scotland and Ireland. He went on to reign for nearly twenty-four years.

On the morning of 2 February 1685 he had an apoplectic fit, dying four days later at Whitehall Palace, which ironically was where his father had been executed on 30 January 1649. He was buried at Westminster Abbey on 14 February 1685 without any pomp or ceremony.

Charles had married Catherine of Braganza, who was born into one of Portugal's most senior noble houses, on 21 May 1662 at Portsmouth. Their marriage produced no children, although Catherine became pregnant on three occasions, each of which resulted in a miscarriage. Although loyal to Catherine in the face of animosity towards her by both courtiers and politicians alike, especially in relation to religious issues and her inability to provide an heir to the throne, Charles had numerous mistresses who, it is said, produced at least a dozen illegitimate children, all of whom he acknowledged. He was succeeded by his brother James, who became James II of England and Ireland and James VII of Scotland.

During his reign Charles had to contend with the Great Plague of London which took place over a period of 18 months during 1665 and 1666, and resulted in the deaths of an estimated 100,000 people, which at the time was nearly a quarter of London's population. Charles, his family and courtiers, left London in July 1665 and went to live in Salisbury, where they remained until February 1666.

On 2 September 1666, in what has become known as the Great Fire of London, a fire broke out in a bakery at Pudding Lane in the City of London. A combination of strong winds, numerous wooden structures and stockpiles of wood, stored in readiness for the forthcoming winter, fanned the flames, which resulted in more than 13,000 houses and nearly 90 churches, including St Paul's Cathedral, being destroyed.

Charles and his brother James took an active part in attempting to extinguish the fires. Despite the fire being no more than an unfortunate and tragic accident, many in society were quick to put the blame on Catholic conspirators with having deliberately started it.

History has looked upon Charles II favourably and he is remembered as one of England's most popular kings, certainly a description with which veteran soldiers who enjoyed the benefits of the Royal Hospital Chelsea would have agreed. Whether he was viewed with the same affection by those from Scotland and Ireland, isn't so clear.

There are numerous statues and memorials that commemorate his name and memory, one of which is a golden statue within the grounds of the Royal Hospital Chelsea, which depicts Charles as an ancient Roman.

Besides the Royal Hospital, he was also the founder of the Royal Observatory as well as a supporter of the Royal Society, and the patron of the renowned architect, Sir Christopher Wren, who constructed the Royal Hospital, and was one of those responsible for rebuilding the City of London in the years following the Great Fire.

What was known as Oak Apple day, was celebrated in England up until around the mid-nineteenth century. This was the date that commemorated the restoration of the English monarchy, 29 May, which had been proclaimed as a public holiday by Parliament in 1660: *'To be for ever kept as a day of thanks giving for our redemption from tyranny and the King's return to his Government, he entering London that day.'*

Although abolished by the Anniversary Days Observance Act 1859, it is still religiously celebrated each year as Founder's Day at the Royal Hospital Chelsea. The name for the celebration is in reference to Charles's escape after the Battle of Worcester on 3 September 1651. To avoid being captured by Cromwell's Roundheads, he hid in the upper branches of an old oak tree that was in Boscobel wood near Boscobel House, and whilst hiding there a Parliamentarian soldier passed directly below where he was, but thankfully did not look up. Lucky that he didn't or otherwise there would have never been any such thing as the Royal Hospital Chelsea, it is doubtful whether Oliver Cromwell would have considered such a building for aged soldiers who had served him.

Charles never forgot the bravery and kindness that Jane Lane displayed in helping him escape to the relative safety of France. On his return to England, Charles showed the extent of his gratitude, by providing her with a pension of £1,000 per year, which was an incredible sum of money at the time. She also received gifts, including a portrait of the king and a lock of his hair, as well as the right for her family to include the three lion's emblem on their coat of arms, an honour in itself.

Lady Jane died on 9 September 1689 at Packington Old Hall, the home that had been built by her husband, Sir Clement Fisher, at Great Packington, near Meriden, in Warwickshire. She was buried in the cemetery of Packington Parish Church.

Richard Hotham was born at York on 5 October 1722, the youngest of five children, but not into a titled family of wealth or importance, just an ordinary one, not poor, but neither were they rich, just somewhere in between. He moved to London sometime during his teenage years to become a hatter's apprentice and in 1743 when he was 21 years of age he married Frances Atkinson, who was the daughter of his employer. This was where his connection with the Royal Hospital Chelsea came from, because it was in the hospital's Wren Chapel where Richard and Frances, were married. How that came to be possible is not known, as neither were from noble families or had any great wealth, privilege or influence in society.

Richard had been taught well. He had listened and watched and asked appropriate questions of his employer, and by 1746 he was sufficiently proficient at his chosen trade to start up his own hat shop in Serle Street, Lincoln's Inn, London. He quickly built up a reputation as a hatter of some note and his business flourished. Before long he had moved to new premises in The Strand, one of the most salubrious business addresses in London.

His wife Frances died in 1760, and within a year Richard had re-married, this time to Barbara Huddart. It was about the same time that he became involved with the East India Company, and his business went to a whole different level. Before long he had a number of ships under his personal control, making him an extremely wealthy young man.

He was knighted in 1768 at the relatively young age of 46. But despite his undoubted wealth and the honour of a knighthood, Richard did not sit back and rest on his laurels. He moved away from the shipping industry and instead ploughed his money into property development. He bought plots of land to build properties on, but also purchased homes as well, including one for himself and his wife in Merton, South London, known as Merton Grove.

His really was a classic example of rags to riches. He went on to become a magistrate in Merton and then became the High Sheriff of Surrey in 1770, and between 1780 and 1784, he was the Member of Parliament for Southwark. A truly remarkable individual who climbed the social ladder all the way to the very top, Sir Richard Hotham died at Bognor in March 1799 and was buried in the small graveyard at St Mary Magdalene Parish Church at South Berstead.

General Sir James Henry Reynett was a British Army officer who had served during the War of the Second Coalition in 1800 as part of the Ferrol expedition, an unsuccessful attempt by the British Army to capture Ferrol from the Spanish. Its appeal was mainly because it was a major Spanish naval base, with a shipyard to build their ships and a dry dock to carry out repairs. In 1808 he was the Deputy Assistant Quartermaster General, during the Peninsular War. Another military position he held was that of Military Secretary to the Duke of Cambridge in 1820, and later the same year he was made the Inspector of Foreign outpatients at the Royal Hospital Chelsea.

By 1831 he had already left the hospital as that was the year that he was appointed as a Groom of the Bedchamber under King William IV, a position in the Royal Household, and one that he held for six years until Queen Victoria took the throne in 1837. His last major post was as the Lieutenant Governor of Jersey between 1847 and 1852. Between 1850 and the time of his death in 1864, he was also the Colonel of the 48th Regiment of Foot. He died in 1864 at the age of 78.

Robert Aris Willmott was born on 30 January 1809 at Bradford, Wiltshire, the son of a local solicitor. In 1819, 10-year-old Robert was admitted to the Merchant Taylors School, a private day school for boys, which at the time was located in the City of London. On leaving there he became a student at Harrow School in 1825, and whilst studying there he was responsible for producing the school's first weekly newspaper in 1828, *The Harrovian*, which is still published today. On 17 February 1834 he began life at Cambridge University, studying at Trinity College, where he was for seven years, finally graduating on 26 May 1841. The following year he was ordained into the Church as a deacon by the Bishop of London, Charles James Blomfield, and just over a year later on 11 June 1843, he became a priest.

His brief connection with the Royal Hospital Chelsea came during a three-month period, between March and June 1845, when he took a service there when he returned to the Church after having been off sick with an unspecified serious illness.

Besides the Church and his religious beliefs, his other great passion was writing, poetry in particular, much of which he had published in books and magazines. His writing spanned from his first publication in 1836, *Conversations at Cambridge*, to 1883, when the second edition of *English Sacred Poetry* was published, twenty years after his death from paralysis on 27 May 1863.

Major General Sir Ronald Bertram Lane was a direct descendent of Jane Lane, through his father, John Newton Lane.

His connection to the Royal Hospital Chelsea stems from his time spent as the hospital's lieutenant governor and secretary between 1905 and 1909. He was a man who had a varied and interesting life, 42 years of which was spent serving in the British Army.

Ronald was born on 19 December 1847 in Kings Bromley, Litchfield, the youngest of ten children. He began his military career at the age of 19 when he was commissioned into the Rifle Brigade as an ensign, the official announcement of which appeared in the edition of the *London Gazette*, dated 1 February 1867.

He saw action during the Zulu War, between 1878 and 1879, and then again in the first Boer War of 1881. During the Battle of Ulundi, the Zulus had

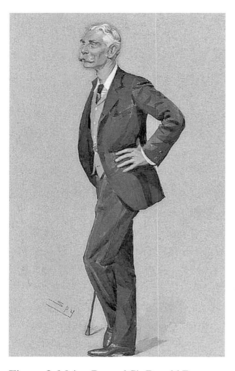

Figure 2: Major General Sir Ronald Bertram Lane.

managed to get to less than 200 yards from the British defensive position and were not showing any signs of being deterred in their efforts. Lane had a bet with one of the war correspondents attached to his regiment in relation to the fighting prowess of the Zulu warriors. As Lane's position worsened an order was given for independent rapid fire in an attempt to quell the Zulu attack. Lane was heard to cheerfully call out to the reporter who was not far from his own location, *'I say …. as we don't seem likely to get out of this square, I'll trouble you to hand over the ten pounds now.'*

He was further promoted over the following years. In 1882 he became aide-de-camp to the Duke of Connaught, as commander of the Guards Brigade in Egypt, and the following year he was made the assistant military secretary in Canada. In 1892 he worked on the headquarters staff in the UK, once again as an assistant military secretary. By 1889 he was aide-de-camp to the Duke of Cambridge and undertook the role of commander-in-chief. He married in 1893, taking as his wife, Augusta Sarah Beaumont, the daughter of John Augustus Beaumont, a developer from Wimbledon in South London.

In 1898 he became the commander of the garrison at Alexandria in Egypt. In December 1901 he moved to Malta where he was appointed commander of the Infantry Brigade. He was so well thought of by his superiors that, in July 1902, he served as Administrator of the Government, during the absence from the island of the Governor, Sir Francis Grenfell.

Between 1903 and 1904, he was appointed as military secretary, which is a British Army appointment, and is held by an officer who holds the rank of major general. The purpose of the role is to advise on policy direction in relation to members of the British Army.

He died at the family home at Carleton Hall in Saxmundham, Suffolk in 1937 at the age of 90. Sir Ronald and Lady Augusta had just one child, George Ronald Lane. Like his father, he was a military man, enlisting at the beginning of the First World War and commissioned as a second lieutenant in the Coldstream Guards. He was further promoted, and at the time of his death on 15 September 1916, during the Battle of the Somme, he was a captain and the adjutant in the 2nd Battalion, Coldstream Guards. He had previously been wounded in 1914. He is buried at the Guards' Cemetery, in the village of Lesboeufs, in the Somme region of France.

I would not like to hazard a guess at what the combined age of all of the in-pensioners who are part of the current group at the Royal Hospital is, but as the minimum age for pensioners to be admitted to this historic institution, is 65, it has to be at least 19,500. Men and women who are in their twilight years and who might be expected to be putting their feet up, sitting in front of a fire, or doing a bit of gentle gardening, are fully immersed in what it takes to be part of the Royal Hospital at Chelsea.

It is highly commendable that a nation not only chooses to look after its elderly veterans in such a way, but that they have chosen to do it for more than 300 years is remarkable. What is apparent if you visit the Royal Hospital Chelsea is how happy and content today's Chelsea Pensioners are. It is quite clear that they do not see it as a right to be a resident there, but more of a privilege and an honour.

The hospital's website describes its own long-term vision, which is to ensure that as an institution it remains relevant to the nation, whilst continuing to be recognised as a place of excellence in the world of care for the elderly. But for this to be achieved it requires both its staff and pensioners to buy in to this ethos by demonstrating the values of, decency, integrity, commitment, comradeship. By conducting themselves in such a manner, they ensure that the high standards expected of them, as the face of the Royal Hospital Chelsea, are maintained and upheld, and that the centuries old traditions can be sustained for the future generations of Chelsea Pensioners.

Chapter 2

The Royal Hospital Chelsea

The building of the Royal Hospital, which for some time after its completion, was still referred to as the Chelsea College, brought with it a lot of attention to the immediate vicinity of Chelsea, which at the time was no more than a village situated on the banks of the River Thames in West London. The site for the Royal Hospital was purchased at a cost of £1,300 from the Royal Society, with the actual build costing an estimated £150,000. The first stone was laid by King Charles II in the presence of a large number of the nation's landed gentry and men and women of nobility.

There is still debate about how the Royal Hospital came into being. Some claim it was down to King Charles, who had been influenced by the Hôtel des Invalides in Paris which had been founded by Louis XIV. Some say it was down to Sir Stephen Fox, who was the first Paymaster General, others place the credit at the feet of actress and mistress of King Charles, Nell Gwynn who, it is said, cajoled the king into building the hospital, by using her womanly charms. She bore him two children, Charles Beauclerk, who was born in 1670 and went on to become the Earl of Burford, and later the Duke of St Albans. Their other son, James Beauclerk, was born the following year in 1671. If her story is the truth behind the hospital's foundation, then sadly she never came to see it reach fruition, as she died in 1687, some five years before it opened.

Chelsea suddenly became a very desirable area in which to live. The hospital's outstanding architecture along with its Royal patronage was more than enough to attract some of London's finest and richest individuals to have new homes built in the area. Many of these exquisite houses were built in the same Dutch-influenced style that Sir Christopher Wren had used to build the Royal Hospital, which had the added attraction of being the first major Royal building since the restoration of the monarchy in 1660.

Chelsea not only attracted the rich and famous to its neighbourhood but also the footpads and highwaymen, who saw the road which ran between Chelsea and the City of London, as an opportunity to unburden some of its new found wealthy residents of their money and jewels, especially during the hours of darkness.

The booklet, *The Royal Hospital at Chelsea* by Lieutenant Colonel Nathaniel Newnham-Davis, which was published in 1912, makes mention of foot patrols that took place every evening until midnight, carried out by some of the hospital's in-pensioners, between St James's Palace and Chelsea. These patrols continued up until 1805. On one occasion the men were attacked, resulting in one of their number being killed and others wounded, after which their assailants made good their escape.

I wondered what Lieutenant Colonel Davis's connection was with the hospital, but apparently there wasn't one. He had served in the British Army during the late 1800s in far off exotic locations, such as South Africa, China and India. By the turn of the century he appears to have left the Army and somehow managed to become a well established and respected restaurant critic in some of London's finest hotels and restaurants, making him an influential figure in the world of cuisine. He wrote for the *Pall Mall Gazette* and was written about and praised in such publications as the *New York Times*. He even wrote three booklets on the subject of food and dining. His first work, *Dinners & Diners (1899), The Gourmet's Guide to Europe (1911)* and *The Gourmet's Guide to London (1914)*.

Over the years the building of dwelling houses as well as industrial premises, continued almost unabated all around the Royal Hospital, with nearly all of the accommodation being acquired by either members of the aristocracy, or the more wealthier in society and, with homes selling at a premium price, the high class reputation of the area continued.

The rules and regulations in relation to the payment of pensions to retired soldiers, which were still paid for directly from the Royal Hospital, meant that individuals in receipt of these payments, had to attend in person to receive their money. They could also be summonsed to the hospital to undergo a medical examination, in relation to their pension. This system was still in place until 1845, meaning that some of the pensioners had to try and find accommodation close to the hospital, which was no easy matter when taking

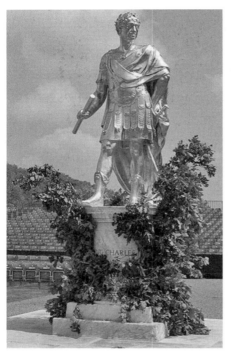

Figure 3: King Charles II.

into account the sums of money in rent that would have been required.

With the rapid increase in the building of homes and other dwellings which took place during the first half of the 1700s, a number of taverns and inns sprang up in some of the less salubrious parts of the district, in the main to accommodate the growing numbers of retired and wounded soldiers who frequented the area, either as visitors or local residents.

The Royal Hospital Chelsea has many wondrous sites to take in, from buildings, to statues, gardens and paintings, all of which help record the long-standing history of this fine establishment. In no particular order here are just a few of them.

King Charles II Statue

The King Charles II statue is in the hospital's central courtyard, which is also known as the Figure Court, and at 7ft 6in in height, is a somewhat larger than life looking character. From a distance, unknowledgeable visitors could be excused for not immediately recognising who the statue represents. At first glance it looks more like a golden painted likeness of Julius Caesar or some other Roman Emperor, rather than King Charles.

The Figure Courts' four-storey East and West wings, contain some of the hospital's living accommodation, on what are referred to as the Long Wards, each of which is 200ft in length with eighteen berths making up each of the wards. In recent times the Chelsea Pensioners' rooms have been upgraded and enlarged on three occasions, first in 1954-55. Again in 1991, and finally in October 2015, when the accommodation was brought into the twenty-first century. Each room has en suite facilities,

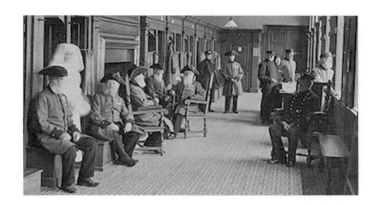

Figure 4: Long Wards at the Royal Hospital Chelsea.

a study area with a desk and chair, along with a large bedroom.

King Charles's statue was cast in copper alloy by Grinling Gibbons. The original version was gilded, but in 1787 it was bronzed. In 2002, as part of the celebrations to mark the Queen's Golden Jubilee, the statue was re-gilded.

Gibbons was born in Rotterdam, Holland on 4 April 1648 and died at the age of 73, on 3 August 1721. He was a Dutch-British sculptor and wood carver. Not a great deal is known of his early life, although it is known that he was living in Deptford, London by about 1667. It is believed that he and his work as an intricate and gifted wood carver, were

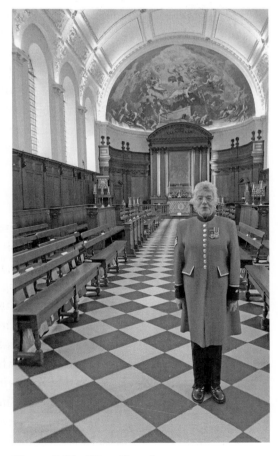

Figure 5: The Wren Chapple.

introduced to King Charles, by the diarist, John Evelyn and Sir Christopher Wren. So impressed was the king by Gibbons' work, that it is he who supposedly gave him his first commission.

The Wren Chapel

Designed by Sir Christopher Wren, the chapel was an addition to the original plan of the Royal Hospital Chelsea and was built between 1681 and 1687. It came about due to King Charles wanting such a place for the pensioners and staff to be able to use for prayer and religious contemplation. It was able to accommodate both the pensioners and staff, which when the hospital first opened its doors, amounted to about 500 people.

The chapel was consecrated in August 1691 and was open daily with compulsory services held twice daily for the resident pensioners. Today there are services only a Sunday morning, Good Friday, Remembrance Sunday, Christmas Eve and Christmas Day. Although couples could be married in the chapel, such ceremonies became less frequent from the mid-1750s onwards and were specifically banned for more than 100 years between 1815 and 1919; funeral services were not held after 1854.

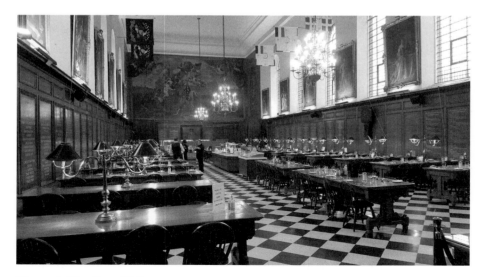

Figure 6: The Great Hall.

The paintings, carvings and stone work within the chapel are a reminder of some of the most highly respected artists of their day including Sir Charles Hopson, one of the leading joiners who went on to become the Royal Hospital's deputy clerk of works between 1691 and 1698. Henry Margetts was responsible for the chapel's plasterwork, whilst the wooden carvings were carried out by William Emmett, Grinling Gibbons and William Morgan. Other influences were the work of Renatus Harris, who was responsible for the chapel's original organ. Other great artists of the day, who were originally involved in the work, were Sebastiano Ricci and his nephew, Marco. Last on the list of artistic luminaries was Ralph Leake, a London silversmith. Little is known about his life other than he worked with Sir Christopher Wren, and King Charles's goldsmith, Sir Robert Vyner.

As an aside, in relation to Ralph Leake, a set of twelve plates made by him in London in about 1700, sold on 23 September 2017, for £36,500.00.

The Great Hall

The original purpose of the Great Hall was for dining, where the pensioners and staff would have their meals. It comprised sixteen long tables, one for each of the hospital's wards, which was where the men lived. There was enough room on each of the tables for twenty-six men. Towards the end of the eighteenth century it was decided that the pensioners and staff would eat their meals on their individual wards. The Great Hall was then used by the pensioners for recreational purposes, and such events as military courts martial and entrance exams for joining the Army.

Throughout the 1800s in particular, it was normal practice if possible, to capture the enemy's flag, colours, banner, standard or eagle. These were the greatest military battle honours it was possible to capture from the enemy. In the Great Hall alone, there are some fifty of these from the armies of many different countries, including Russia, China, France, Arabic, America, Malta, Holland, and Ceylon. There is also a French Eagle that was captured from the French 45th Regiment during the Battle of Waterloo on 18 June 1815 by Sergeant Ewart of the Scots Greys.

In the Wren Chapel there are some forty-three captured flags and standards along with another twelve Eagles. One of these, the Eagle of the 39th French Regiment, wasn't won in battle, but found in the River Ceira in Portugal, on 15 June 1811, whilst another, that of the 13th French Regiment, was found in the Retiro, Madrid in August 1812.

In 1852 the Great Hall was chosen as the location for the lying in state of the body of Arthur Wellesley, the 1st Duke of Wellington, prior to his funeral at St Paul's Cathedral in the City of London.

Some of the first visitors to the Great Hall during Wellington's lying in state, were Queen Victoria, accompanied by Prince Albert, the Prince of Wales and the Princess Royal. After the Royal guests had paid their respects, the hospital's own veterans, some of whom had no doubt served under Wellington, were allowed in to see him. Next came those dignitaries who had been provided with a ticket by the Lord Chamberlain's office. Last but by no means least, and for a four-day period, members of the public were admitted without tickets. So great was the demand for a last glimpse of the beloved Wellington, that a crush ensued as the crowds rushed in resulting in the deaths of several people.

The table on which his coffin was placed is still in use today in the Great Hall. While he was lying in state somebody broke into the chapel via the roof and stole a gilt bronze or golden eagle, the staff it was attached to, and a banner. The staff was found nearby, but there was no trace of the eagle or banner. The eagle had been captured by the 87th Regiment of Foot (Royal Irish Fusiliers) at the Battle of Barrosa, near Cadiz in Spain on 5 March 1811.

The duke, who had twice been the British Prime Minister between 1828 and 1834, was better known for his defeat of Napoleon at the Battle of Waterloo in 1815, and remains one of the nation's best loved military heroes. He died from what is believed to have been a stroke aged 83, at Walmer Castle in Kent, on 14 September 1852. His final resting place is at St Paul's Cathedral in the City of London.

The original use of the hall was reinstated in 1955 and remains the same to this day. Numerous portraits of past kings and queens, murals and period paintings adorn the walls of the Great Hall, some of which date back to the late 1600s.

Ranelagh Gardens

Today Ranelagh Gardens form part of the magnificent grounds of the Royal Hospital Chelsea, but that wasn't always the case. Today's gardens are the work of Mr John Gibson, and were designed in about 1860. They were originally the gardens of Ranelagh House, a property built in 1688–1689, by Solomon Rieti, whose humble beginnings began as an Italian Jewish immigrant. He built the property for the Earl of Ranelagh, who was the Treasurer of the Royal Hospital between 1685 and 1702. The gardens of the property immediately adjoined the hospital.

Sir Thomas Robinson, a Member of Parliament for Morpeth, the owner of the Theatre Royal Drury Lane, and a syndicate of other interested parties, purchased Ranelagh House and its grounds in 1741. The gardens were opened to the public the following year and, because of the location in fashionable Chelsea, attracted large crowds of people who were more than happy to pay the entrance charge of two shillings and six pence. It is said that Ranelagh Gardens introduced the masquerade to a much wider audience of society, which had previously been the sole domain of the elite.

Ranelagh House was demolished in 1805, and although the gardens remained, they were redesigned by John Gibson in about 1860. Fulham Football Club played their home matches there for two years between 1886–1888, when it was known as the Ranelagh Ground. Besides today being part of the Royal Hospital Chelsea, it is also the location for the world-famous Chelsea Flower Show, which takes place there every year in May, and has done so since 1913.

Over the years the Royal Hospital Chelsea has seen many changes, whether in the shape of improvements to the facility, the staff who have worked there or the pensioners fulfilling the purpose it was built for, 325 years later they are a testimony to what it has achieved over such a long period of time. Let's hope that it is still in place in another 325 years time, not because of war or conflicts, but just so that old soldiers in the twilight of their years have such a place where they can live and be cared for.

Courts Martial

During the late 1700s and early 1800s numerous courts martial took place at the Royal Hospital Chelsea, of senior British Army officers, these hearings being held mainly in the hospital's Great Hall. Here are the details of just a few of them. All of the trials that I have come across have been in relation to officers only. One of these cases includes an act of mutiny where the officer concerned was found guilty of the offence, his punishment was, to be 'cashiered', which in layman's terms means that he was discharged or sacked from the Army. When considering how severe a punishment this was, take into account that until 1998, when Section 21 (5) of the Human Rights Act completely abolished the death penalty throughout the United Kingdom, the maximum punishment for anybody who committed an act of mutiny whilst serving in the British Armed Forces, was death, as per the conditions of the Army Act 1955.

The General Court Martial of : **Major Andrew Armstrong:** of the 11th (North Devonshire) Regiment of Foot, took place on Saturday, 22 June 1799.

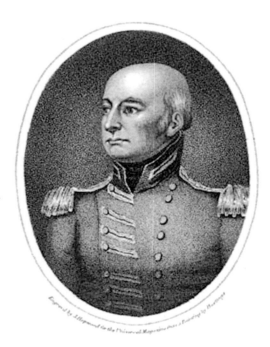

The General Court Martial of: **Captain John Flory Howard:**, of the Royal Regiment of Horse Guards in November 1798.

The General Court Martial of: **Major General Burton:**, of the 3rd Regiment of Foot, took place between Friday 6 and Monday, 9 January 1804.

The General Court Martial of: **Lieutenant General John Whitelocke:**, who had previously been the Commander–in–Chief of British Forces in South America, took place in the Great Hall at the Royal Hospital Chelsea on Thursday, 28 January 1808, and continued by adjournment until Friday, 18 March.

Figure 7: Lieutenant General John Whitelocke.

Lieutenant General John Whitelocke had attempted to wrest back control of Buenos Aires, in Argentina, following the surrender of General Beresford, but was unsuccessful and was forced to withdraw. Soon afterwards, he returned to England, not to be met with a warm homecoming, but where he faced a court martial and, on being found guilty as charged, he was cashiered from the Army for his failure.

The two charges that he faced were as follows:

First charge:

That whilst in Buenos Aires, pursued measure ill calculated to facilitate that conquest, that when the Spanish Commander had shown such symptoms of a disposition to treat, as to express a desire to communicate with Major General Gower, the second in command, upon the subject of terms, the said Lieutenant General Whitelocke, did return a message, in which he demanded, amongst other articles, the surrender of all persons holding civil offices in the Government of Buenos Aires as prisoners of war: that the said Lieutenant General Whitelocke in making such an offensive and unusual demand, tended to exasperate the inhabitants of Buen, to produce and encourage a spirit of resistance to His Majesty's arms, to exclude the hope of an amicable accommodation, and to increase the difficulties of the service with which he was intrusted, acted in a manner unbecoming his duty as an officer, prejudicial to military discipline, and contrary to the articles of war.

Second charge:

That the said Lieutenant General Whitelocke, after the landing of troops at Ensenada, and during the march from thence to the town of Buenos Aires, did not make the military agreements best calculated to ensure the success of his operations against the town, and that having known, previously to his attack upon the town of Buenos Aires upon the 5ᵗʰ July 1807, as appears from his public disaster of the 5ᵗʰ July, that the enemy meant to occupy the roofs of the houses, he did nevertheless, in the said attack, divide his forces into several Brigades and parts, and ordered the whole to be unloaded, and no tiring to be permitted on any account; and, under this order, to march into the principal streets of the town unprovided with proper and sufficient means for forcing the barricades, whereby the troops were unnecessarily exposed to destruction, without the possibility of making effective opposition; such conduct betraying great professional incapacity on the part of the said Lieutenant General Whitelocke, tending to lessen the confidence of the troops in the judgement of their officers, being derogatory to the honour of His Majesty's arms, contrary to his duty as an officer, prejudicial to good order and military discipline, contrary to the articles of war.

So serious was the case that there were twenty-two members of the court, which included the Judge Advocate, the Hon. Richard Ryder, six generals and fourteen lieutenant generals. A less formidable band of brothers it would have been harder to muster, and whether or not John Whitelocke felt intimidated by their very presence in the hospital's Great Hall, the answer to which is not known, they would have certainly presented themselves so, intentionally or otherwise, as they sat in front of the accused in their full military regalia.

The Judge Advocate, Mr Ryder, in opening the court martial, enquired of Lieutenant General Whitelocke as to whether he was guilty or not guilty, to which he replied, 'Not Guilty'.

His opening address to the members of the court, who would ultimately determine Whitelocke's fate, included the following summation, his words echoed throughout the Great Hall for all to hear:

The reduction of the province of Buenos Aires, has totally failed. That it failed with the lamentable loss of a large proportion of the gallant army engaged in it, that it failed not only in accomplishing its object, but that it ended in the absolute surrender of those valuable advantages which the valour of the British troops, under another commander, had previously acquired in the important post of Monte Video.

As he continued with his opening address it became very apparent that his diatribe, which was ultimately aimed at Lieutenant General Whitelocke, was not only driven by the large number of soldiers, good men and loyal servants of the crown who had lost their lives in the subsequent fighting, but the lost opportunity of discovering new markets for the nation's manufacturers and merchants to sell their wares to what was described as: '*The rude wants of countries emerging from barbarism, or the artificial and increasing demands of luxury and refinement in those remote quarters of the globe.*'

Mr Ryder also made reference to the military embarrassment that such a defeat had caused to the nation.

The disappointment too has been cruelly embittered by the disgrace which such a failure under the circumstances have attached to the British Arms. A diminution of our military fame must be ever felt as a great national calamity, but at no period so severely as in this crisis of the world, when our military character is become more essential than ever, not merely our honour or our glory, but for the independence, the liberties, the existence of Great Britain.'

The court martial papers for the case stretched to some 830 pages. In the first instance, the trial lasted for twenty-nine consecutive days, until Monday, 7 March. It re-commenced on Monday, 14 March, and then continued on for a further five days, finally coming to an end on Friday, 18 March.

On being found guilty of two of the charges against him, the following sentence was announced:

The Court Martial having dully considered the evidence given in support of the charges against the prisoner, Lieutenant General Whitelocke, his defence, and the evidence he has adduced, are of opinion, that he is guilty of the whole of the said charges, with the exception of that part of the second charge which relates to the order that 'the columns should be unloaded, and that no firing should be permitted on any account.'

The Court are anxious that it may be distinctly understood, that they attach no censure whatever to the precautions taken to prevent unnecessary firing during the advance of the troops to the proposed points of attack, and do therefore acquit Lieutenant General Whitelocke of that part of the said charge.

The Court adjudge, that the said Lieutenant General Whitelocke be cashiered, and declared totally unfit, and unworthy, to serve his Majesty in any Military capacity whatever.

King George III himself had confirmed the decision, and such was his displeasure over the matter that he directed that details of the court martial should be read out to every regiment in his Army, and entered in every Regimental Orderly Book, with a view to its becoming a lasting reminder to all officers to not act in a similar way in the future.

It would appear that Lieutenant General Whitelocke had already been dammed before the court martial had even begun. It could be argued that the loss of potentially new commercial openings, much sought after by the government and the nation's merchants, as well as the perceived military embarrassment, were the driving force behind this court martial. Somebody had to pay, there had to be somebody to blame, and unfortunately for Lieutenant General Whitelocke, it was him.

After leaving the Army he went to live at Hall Barn Park at Beaconsfield in Buckinghamshire, where he died on 23 October 1833.

Another General Court Martial took place in the Great Hall of the Royal Hospital Chelsea on (3 April 1811) Tuesday, 11 May 1811, this time the man facing trial was **Lieutenant Colonel George Johnston**, of the 102nd Regiment of Foot, late of the New South Wales Corps, on a charge of Mutiny, when he was Major George Johnston, captain of the said Corps, which was then under his command and stationed in Sydney, New South Wales.

His offence, was that on 26 January 1808, he committed an act of mutiny by deposing William Bligh, Esq. F.R.S, who was then a Captain in His Majesty's Navy, Captain General and the Governor-in-Chief of the territory of New South Wales, and took his place as the Governor of New South Wales. This became known as the Rum Rebellion.

The charge of mutiny was read out to the court:

That Lieutenant Colonel George Johnston, Major as aforesaid, did on or about the 26th day of January 1808, at Sydney, in the colony of New South Wales, begin, excite, cause and join in a mutiny by putting himself at the head of the New South Wales Corps, then under his command and doing duty in the colony and seizing and causing to be seized and arrested, and imprisoning and causing to be imprisoned, by means of the above mentioned military force, the person of William Bligh, Esq. then

Captain General and Governor in Chief in and over the territory of New South Wales.

This was an enormous case with twenty-two witnesses being called for the Crown, with a further eighteen witnesses being called in support of Lieutenant Colonel Johnston.

The man in charge of the proceedings, who was appointed as its President, was Lieutenant General William Keppel, Colonel of His Majesty's 67th South Hampshire Regiment of Foot. The Judge Advocate General in the trial, was the Right Hon. Charles Manners Sutton, who began the proceedings by asking Lieutenant Colonel Johnston if he wished to plead guilty or not guilty to the charge which was preferred against him. He replied, 'Not guilty'.

It was an unusual case as in so far as the offence that the defendant had been charged with, had allegedly taken place, some three years earlier. Even some of the court members were uncomfortable about this particular aspect of the case, and made their feelings known to the Judge Advocate. The main bone of contention was the fact that the court was only legally allowed to hear a case where the incident which had led to the trial had taken place less than three years earlier. In this particular matter the incident had taken place more than three years earlier. Some members of the court understandably questioned the legality of the trial. The Judge Advocate answered in these terms, based as he stated, on his understanding of the law:

No trial shall take place where the facts upon the charge bear date more than three years before the issuing of the warrant for holding the Court Martial, unless some manifest impediment has arisen. Therefore, if more than three years has elapsed, to legalise the holding of a Court Martial, some manifest impediment must have arisen, and that manifest impediment must be stated in order to enable the Court to form a judgement upon it; the Court cannot form that judgement until they hear the evidence; the Court therefore proceed upon the trial by calling evidence: and the only question now is, whether the Court will invert the natural order of things by calling that evidence first, or whether they will let it come on its ordinary and natural course.

The Judge Advocate continued with his interpretation of the law. The way he saw it was that questions had to be asked of witnesses so that the court could establish if there were in fact any impediments which had prevented an earlier hearing of the evidence. Once this had been established, they would then be able to determine whether the case against Lieutenant Colonel Johnston could continue.

Two of the court members were still not happy with this answer and pushed the Judge Advocate further on the matter of the three-year rule, whilst the other, asked whether or not the question could be asked of Captain Bligh. This request was declined by the Judge Advocate, who said there would be no point in asking such a question as the case was before them because it had been so ordered by the Crown and not because of any one individual.

Lieutenant Colonel Johnston was found guilty of mutiny and was cashiered from the Army, after what had been a distinguished military career. He had been an officer in the Marines during the American Revolutionary War, also known as the American War of Independence, that lasted between 1775 and 1783, and which saw Great Britain pitted against the thirteen colonies of the newly formed United States of America, which had declared independence. He also served in the East Indies, where he fought against the French, and volunteered to be part of the crew that travelled as part of the First Fleet to New South Wales in Australia.

In May 1813 he returned to New South Wales; no longer a military man, he became a farmer in the Annandale area of Sydney. In November 1814 he married Esther Abrahams at St John's Church, in Parramatta, by which time he was 50 years of age.

Ceremonies

Two ceremonies worthy of note include one that is some 300 years old and another that has it roots as recently as 1949. The first is the Ceremony of the Christmas Cheeses, an annual event, which not surprisingly takes place over the Christmas period, and has done so since the beginning of the hospital's history in 1692. At the time, the authorities of the Royal Hospital Chelsea, approached a local cheesemonger and asked them to provide its in-pensioners with sufficient cheese to see them through the Christmas period. This they willingly did and it has since become a tradition at the hospital.

Each year since 1961 the Dairy Council of the United Kingdom has organised a special ceremony which takes place at the hospital, where they provide the residents with cheese from all around the country. One of the veterans is selected to cut the ceremonial cheese with a sword and distribute it amongst the hospital's other patients over the Christmas period.

The Christmas Cake Ceremony is another annual event which takes place each year at the Royal Hospital Chelsea and signifies the lasting friendship which exists between Australia and the United Kingdom. It is a ceremony which dates back to 1949 when representatives of the Australian Returned and Services League, an organisation equivalent to the Royal British Legion, present a cake to the pensioners at the Royal Hospital Chelsea, during the festive period, with the ceremony taking place in the Great Hall. A different state of Australia gets to present the cake each year. As with the Ceremony of the Christmas Cake, a Chelsea Pensioner is selected to cut the cake with a sword. A number of Chelsea Pensioners have served with the Australian forces in some capacity over the years.

Singora Cannon

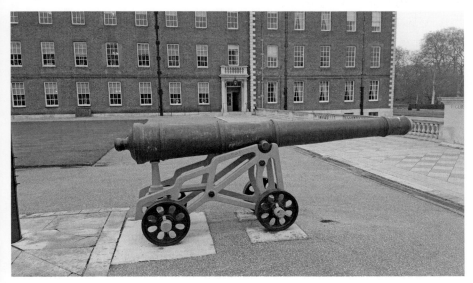

The Singora Cannon sits prominently in the grounds of the Figure Court at the Royal Hospital Chelsea. The cannon, which dates back nearly 400 years is believed to have been made in 1623, for the Sultanate of Singora, a heavily fortified port city in southern Thailand and which today has the name of Songkhla. The cannon bears the seal of the Sultan Sulaiman and was originally captured by the Siamese in 1680. It remained with them until the Siamese-Burmese War of 1765-1767, when it was captured by the Burmese and transported back to Burma as a trophy, where it remained for well over a hundred years until the Third Anglo-Burmese War which took place between 7 and 29 November 1885, when it was captured by the British and shipped back to England. Following the war, Burma in its entirety, came under the rule of the British Raj as a province of India.

On 27 November 1956 her Majesty Queen Elizabeth II, was the guest of honour at a dinner given by the Army Council and the Army, in the ancient and resplendent surroundings of the Great Hall at the Royal Hospital Chelsea.

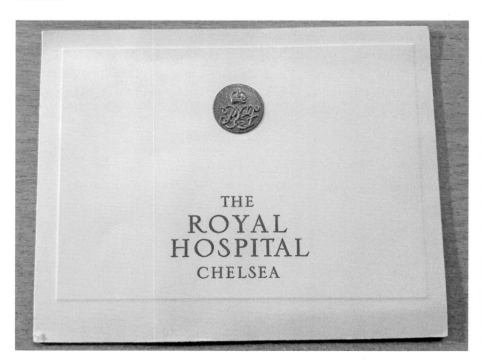

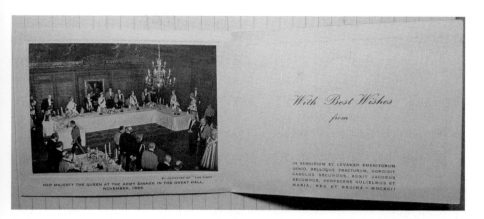

HER MAJESTY THE QUEEN AT THE ARMY DINNER IN THE GREAT HALL,
NOVEMBER, 1956.

With Best Wishes
from

IN SUBSIDIUM ET LEVAMEN EMERITORUM
SENIO, BELLOQUE FRACTORUM, CONDIDIT
CAROLUS SECUNDUS, AUXIT JACOBUS
SECUNDUS, PERFECERE GULIELMUS ET
MARIA, REX ET REGINA — MDCXCII

The Queen was accompanied by other members of the Royal family. Each regiment and corps of the British Army was represented by its colonel, and senior officers from the liaison staffs in London attended as representatives of the Commonwealth.

Her Majesty took her place at the centre of the top table. Sitting immediately to her right were, Mr John Hare, Secretary of State for War; Queen Elizabeth the Queen Mother; Field Marshal Lord Ironside; the Duke of Gloucester; the Duchess of Kent and Field Marshal Sir Claude Auchinleck. To the left were: Field Marshal Sir Gerald Templer, Chief of the Imperial General Staff; Princess Margaret; Field Marshal Lord Alanbrooke; the Duchess of Gloucester and the Princess Royal.

Chapter 3

The Chelsea Pensioners

The world-famous Chelsea Pensioners have been a part of British history since the Royal Hospital, which is a 66-acre site situated in Chelsea, first opened on 4 February 1692, when ninety-nine pensioners walked through the hospital's doors into history. These were followed on 28 March 1692 by a further 377, making a grand total of 476. The hospital was originally intended for only 412 residents.

Originally, the plans drawn up by Sir Christopher Wren only included a single quadrangle, but before the work on the hospital had even begun, he realised that the number of buildings he had allowed for, would not be sufficient to cater for the number of intended pensioners, so Wren added two further quadrangles to his original design. It was 1686 when the construction of the hospital was finally approved and the building work commenced.

Part of the money for the building was acquired by deductions from soldiers' Army pay. This practice of obtaining funds to finance the continued existence of the hospital remained in place until 1847, when the main funding then became the responsibility of the Ministry of Defence, which they achieved by what is called, 'Grant in Aid.'

The hospital was the brain child of King Charles II and had been founded by him ten years earlier in 1682 as a retreat for wounded veterans, but the idea for providing veterans with a home rather than paying them a pension, had French roots in the shape of *Les Invalides* in Paris. This had come from King Louis XIV, when he issued an order dated 24 November 1670 for the building of a hospital and a home for elderly and unwell soldiers referred to as *hôpital des invalids*. The hospital was designed and built by the respected French architect, Libéral Bruant. It took six years to complete and opened in 1676, although it was then decided that the veterans residing there required a chapel for prayer, which was completed in 1679 with Jules

Hardouin-Mansart assisting the by now aging Bruant who died before its completion on 22 November 1697. Despite his death the building of the chapel was completed to Bruant's original design.

King Charles never lived to see his dream come true. He died aged 54 on 6 February 1685, four days after suffering what was interpreted as an apoplectic fit, and having no legitimate heir, was succeeded by his brother, James II. His reign was a relatively short one, lasting from 6 February 1685 until 11 December 1688, when he was deemed to have abdicated after his nephew and son-in-law William of Orange brought an invading army over from the Dutch Republic in what is often referred to as the Glorious Revolution of 1688. James fled to France and his eldest daughter, Mary, who was a Protestant, and her husband William III took the English crown.

It was during William's reign that the Royal Hospital was finally completed, so that before it had even opened its doors, three different monarchs had sat on the English throne, thankfully none of them bringing its building to a halt. In fact, King William and Queen Mary were so supportive of the idea that they instigated army pensions in 1689, some three years before the Royal Hospital had actually opened its doors. These pensions were available to all former soldiers who had been injured during their military service, or who had served their king and country for more than 20 years.

Some of the first residents at the hospital were veterans of the Battle of Sedgemoor which took place on 6 July 1685 at Westonzoyland near Bridgwater in Somerset, between the royal army of James II and the rebel army of James Scott, 1st Duke of Monmouth.

All Army pensions were the responsibility of the Royal Hospital until as recently as 1955. This was the reason for the variation of titles given to those in receipt of such pensions. Those who were resident in the Royal Hospital and enjoyed the benefits of doing so were referred to as in-pensioners, but to do so meant they had to surrender their army pension to the hospital in lieu of being fed and provided with a roof over their heads. Those who lived in towns, villages and cities up and down the country and who were in receipt of their army pension, were classed as out-pensioners. Once the payment of army pensions stopped being the responsibility of the hospital, the term out-pensioner, became somewhat redundant, but then over time, so did use of the phrase in-pensioner.

The Royal Hospital Chelsea is governed by a Board of Commissioners, who have a responsibility to move it forward in a positive way, whilst at the same time ensuring that it remains as a retirement and nursing home for former members of the British Army.

Before a former soldier can apply to become a resident he has to fulfil qualifying criteria. Firstly, they must have reached their sixty-fifth birthday, have at least twenty-two years Army service, have no dependent wife or children and be free and able to live on what are referred to as the hospital's Long Wards. They have to have previously served in the British Army as a soldier or non-commissioned officer. Former army officers can also be admitted to the hospital, but they must have served in the 'other ranks' for a minimum of twelve years, or have been awarded a disability pension whilst serving in the ranks.

On entering the hospital, a pensioner has to surrender his army pension and in return is provided with their own en suite private room on one of the wards and allocated to one of the companies. Their meals are paid for, they are provided with the regulation hospital clothing and uniforms as well as full medical care. If a pensioner becomes ill, they are moved into the hospital's infirmary, which is a state of the art facility.

The pensioner's rooms were not always so spacious. Up until the 1950s they were just 6ft square in size, and the most recent improvements were completed in 2015. The hospital also provides excellent social amenities as well as allotments for pensioners with green fingers or lawn bowls for the more energetic.

The pensioners are provided with two distinct uniforms, or what are referred to as the 'scarlets' or 'blues'. The blue uniforms are usually worn when in the hospital grounds or when out and about in the surrounding area. When travelling further afield, the pensioners are expected to wear the scarlet long coats, which are also worn for ceremonial duties, along with the easy recognisable tricorne hats. At all other times a black peaked hat is worn, which is known as a shako, a popular military style of headdress of the early 1800s, and which originated from the Hungarian name, csako, although these tended to be much taller in height. When pensioners are wearing their uniforms they display the insignia of the rank that they had reached whilst serving in the British Army. They also wear the medals they were awarded, along with any other recognised insignia such as SAS jump wings or Parachute Regiment jump wings.

Non-commissioned officers from the rank of lance corporal to staff sergeant, display stripes on their uniforms, and warrant officers and above, wear either a crown or a coat of arms badge. Until 1843 all men, no matter what their rank, wore breeches. It was only after this time that trousers became part of the uniform. A new style of trousers was issued in 1961 – dark-blue tweed adorned with a thin scarlet stripe which ran down the outer seam of each leg. This is the same style of trousers that both the male and female Chelsea Pensioners wear today.

The Blues – In 1707 Pensioners were issued with a dark-blue coloured 'greatcoat', because before this time many of them only had one set of clothes, so it helped to keep them warm in the winter. This was eventually replaced with the double-breasted blue jacket, which is still in use today and is worn all year round. Medals are not worn on the 'blues' as the uniform is casual dress and is for everyday wear. Instead medal ribbons adorn the left chest area jacket. Medals are worn for formal occasions when the 'scarlet' uniform is worn.

The shako peaked cap previously mentioned was first introduced in 1843, and was very similar in design to what was worn with the Army uniform of the time. They are still worn today and are embroidered with the letters RH, the initials of the Royal Hospital. They are a very popular part of the uniform for the pensioners; besides being seen as being more practical, they are also said to be more comfortable to wear than the tricorns.

The Scarlets

The long scarlet coat of the Chelsea Pensioners has become an iconic item of clothing, which is recognised the world over as being quintessentially British. It can be worn with either the everyday shako cap, or the ceremonial tricorne hat, which along with white gloves, is worn for ceremonial occasions, when a member of the Royal family is present.

Each coat is adorned with nine buttons all of which are engraved with the initials RCI. This stands for the Royal Corps of Invalids, a unit of which

Chelsea Pensioners were once a part. Their officer in charge is still referred to as the Captain of Invalids.

The buttons used to be made of brass, but haven't been so since 1959, and although Chelsea Pensioners are the epitome of the meaning of the word, tradition, they are more than happy with the replacement anodised buttons, which do not require polishing.

The tricorne hat has originated, not as some might believe by design, but operational necessity. Originally, they were felt hats with a rim all the way round, which during battle could be something of a hindrance, especially if it was raining. It was also a form of headdress that was a popular amongst the male civilian population, by both commoner and aristocracy alike, during the eighteenth century, although it was falling out of favour by 1800. Strangely enough during the time that the hat was in fashion, it was actually referred to as a Cocked Hat. It didn't acquire the name Tricorne, until the mid-1800s.

Elsewhere in this book is the story of Mrs Christian Davis who was admitted to the Royal Hospital Chelsea in the early 1700s. In April 2007 an official announcement was made explaining that women were to be permitted as in-pensioners but this didn't actually take place for a further two years, when on 12 March 2009, Dorothy Hughes and Winifred Phillips joined the pensioners' ranks at the hospital. The reason for the delay between the announcement and Winifred actually becoming a pensioner, was due to the time it took to raise the money needed to carry out extensive redevelopment at the hospital, including the installation of female bathrooms and lavatories.

Winifred was born in Ilford in 1926. In 1948 she enlisted in the Auxiliary Territorial Service (ATS), which was the women's branch of the British Army during the Second World War, before it was disbanded on 1 February 1949, at which time it was merged into the Women's Royal Army Corps. Whilst serving with the ATS, Winifred was stationed in Egypt, and when the change came she then spent the next twenty-two years serving with the Women's Royal Army Corps in Singapore, Cyprus, and Egypt, finishing at the rank of Warrant Officer Class 2.

Years after her retirement she eventually got around to approaching the hospital to ask about being admitted as a pensioner. It turned out that the reason women hadn't been admitted to the hospital prior to this was because those who made such decisions at the time, simply hadn't considered such an eventuality.

As a 16-year-old girl, Winifred was training to be a nursery nurse when she met and fell in love with George Wheeler, who was 19 and a trainee wireless operator in the RAF. In 1943 and with his training completed, he was sent on bombing missions to Germany from RAF Wyton in Cambridgeshire. They kept in touch, but one day in 1944 the Avro Lancaster Bomber he was on, went missing.

A check of the Commonwealth War Graves Commission website, records that a total of twenty men with the name George Wheeler were killed during the Second World War. Of these four were members of the Royal Air Force Volunteer Reserve. Only one of these was buried in Germany and that was Sergeant 1393912 George Wheeler of No.83 Squadron, who died on 20 February 1944, and is buried at the Berlin 1939–1945 War Cemetery. George's Squadron were part of No.8 Pathfinder Force, whose job was as a marker unit for the main force of bomber command.

Winifred was admitted to the hospital in 2009 when she was 82 years of age. She wrote two books during her time spent as an in-pensioner. The first was published in 2010 entitled, *My Journey to Becoming the First Lady Chelsea Pensioner* and in 2013 she brought out *Mum's Army: Love and Adventure from the NAAFI to Civvy Street*.

Winifred passed away on 14 February 2016 aged 89. Sadly, on average one pensioner each week dies, on such occasions this is referred to as the 'Last Posting'. If we accept this figure as an accurate average of Chelsea in-pensioners who have died whilst they were residents of the Royal Hospital, this means that up to and including November 2017, and taking into account the 300 men and women who are current incumbents, there have been a total of at least 18,208 pensioners who have lived at the hospital during the time of its existence.

Dorothy Hughes enlisted in the British Army in 1941, eventually becoming part of the 450th Heavy Artillery Battery in the London Division. As the war slowly drew to a close, Dorothy's Battery was sent to Dover to help combat the rising threat of the German V-1 rockets coming in over the Kent coastline en route to London.

Dorothy later transferred to the Army Operational Research Group where she helped develop fuses for the shells that were used to try and bring down the V2 Rockets. She was discharged from the Army in 1946 at the rank of sergeant and started a new life in teaching.

At the time of writing this chapter of the book (October 2017) Dorothy was still an in-pensioner at the Royal Hospital Chelsea.

Chapter 4

Sir Christopher Wren and Sir Stephen Fox

It wouldn't be appropriate to write a book on the Royal Hospital Chelsea, and not include something about Sir Christopher Wren, who was responsible for the design and building of the hospital, and Sir Stephen Fox, who was commissioned by King Charles II to find the money that would pay for it.

Christopher Wren was born on 30 October 1632 in Wiltshire. Although he had four sisters, he was the only surviving son of Christopher Wren and Mary Cox, the only child of the Wiltshire

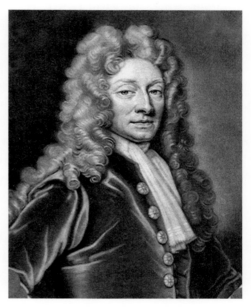

Figure 8: Sir Christopher Wren.

squire, Robert Cox. On his death Mary inherited her father's estate, making the family more than financially secure. At the time of his son's birth Christopher senior was the Rector at East Knoyle and in March 1635 he became the Dean of Windsor by Royal appointment. In those early years of his life he was taught by his father as well as a private tutor, the Reverend William Shepherd, a local clergyman. Because of his father's position, Christopher and the rest of his family would spend some of his time at home in East Knoyle and part of the time in Windsor.

When he was 18 years of age he attended Wadham College, Oxford University. There he was taught Latin and Science, and first exposed to the importance which mathematics played in the world. His teacher was

Dr William Holder, who also happened to be his brother-in-law, having married Christopher's elder sister Susan in 1643.

After a year of prolonged and continuous study, Christopher graduated with a BA in his studies of maths and science and in 1653, an MA. He also showed himself to be a gifted artist. He continued his studies at All Souls College, Oxford. By the time he was 25 years of age, he had been appointed as a Professor of Astronomy at the highly respected Gresham College in London, where he gave weekly lectures in both English and Latin, free of charge, to anybody who wished to attend. It was a reasonably well-paid position and came with a set of rooms for his accommodation and study.

He very quickly became a prominent and respected figure in the scientific community, and from 1660 onwards would regularly meet up with other like minded and learned individuals in the field of science and he very soon came to the attention of the king. In 1662 Charles II gave the Society of London for Improving Natural Knowledge, of which Wren was a founding member, its royal charter. The previous year Wren had been elected as the Savilian Professor of Astronomy at Oxford University, where he would stay for the following seven years, until he was appointed to the position of Surveyor of Works to King Charles in 1669.

For a man to have such a wide knowledge of so many different topics, to the extremely high standard which Wren did, was beyond remarkable, it bordered on being almost unbelievable. The Royal Society records that his achievements were as varied as they were many, and included, astronomy, optics, finding longitude at sea, cosmology (the study of the origin, evolution and eventual fate of the universe) a term which had only been first used in English in 1656, mechanics, microscopy, surveying, medicine and meteorology. As if that wasn't enough for one man to have learned to such a high degree of knowledge, he observed, measured, dissected, built models, made inventions as well as improved numerous instruments that were already in existence.

Most men would be satisfied to be so highly knowledgeable in just one such discipline, let alone so many, yet today when Sir Christopher Wren's name is mentioned, it is for architecture that he is best remembered, in particular for his re-building of St Paul's Cathedral after the Great Fire of London in 1665, greatly inspired no doubt by the architecture in Paris, which he had visited earlier in the year.

It has some worth to reflect on the costs involved in such an undertaking as that of the Royal Hospital Chelsea, and how, after it had opened its doors to veteran British soldiers, the continued running costs of housing, clothing and feeding both the pensioners who were to live there and the staff who were to look after them, were to be met. In erecting the building, monies needed to be found for the costs of the labour and materials, as well as the wages of the staff, and a day on day figure for each of the pensioners who lived there.

The Royal Hospital Chelsea was the first large project which Wren designed and took ten years to build, starting in 1682 by which time Wren was 50 years of age. It opened its doors to accept its first Chelsea Pensioners in February 1692. It was as if Wren's life, knowledge and ability had been fine tuned to arrive at that very point in time, to provide him with the skill and know-how to design and erect the Royal Hospital Chelsea.

An interesting point to finish on is that all of Wren's large scale, secular, architectural commissions, are from after 1680.

Stephen Fox was born on 27 March 1627 in Farley, Wiltshire, the same county as Christopher Wren. His father was a Yeoman farmer, a commoner who cultivated his own land, which meant that Stephen had not experienced an overly affluent family upbringing. His achievements in adult life were the result of a university education, making what he went on to achieve in society, a truly remarkable feat.

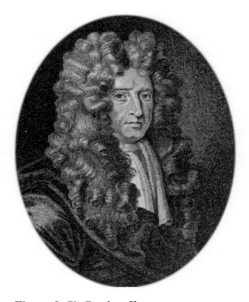

Besides being the man whom King Charles relied upon to find the required funding to make his dream of a Royal Hospital a reality, he was also the commander at the hospital between 1691 to 1703, after which time he left to become a director at the Greenwich Hospital.

Sir Stephen not only served under Charles II, but James II and William III. His loyalty to

Figure 9: Sir Stephen Fox.

the Crown was second to none. When Charles II escaped to Europe on 16 October 1651, by boat from Shoreham-on-Sea, after his defeat at the Battle of Worcester, one of his companions was Sir Stephen. When the restored monarch returned to England in 1660 Sir Stephen returned with him and for his loyalty he was appointed to the lucrative position of Clerk of the Green Cloth, in the Royal Household, which involved organising royal journeys and the day to day administration of the royal household. He was also made the Paymaster of the Forces, a position in the British Government, which was established in 1661 which meant he was responsible in part for the financing of the British Army. This was a post he held on two occasions. First between 1661 and 1676 and 1679 and 1680.

In 1661 he also embarked on a career in English politics which would continue until his death on 28 October 1716, aged 89. During his first term of office he was knighted for his years of loyalty by King Charles II.

In 1661 to 1679, he served as the MP for Salisbury; in 1679 as the MP for Westminster; from 1685 to 1689 he was MP for Salisbury; from 1691 to 1698 he was MP for Westminster; from 1699 to 1702 was MP for Cricklade and between 1714 and 1715 for the Parliamentary constituency of Salisbury.

Stephen Fox was a resourceful man who managed to raise £13,000 for the building of the Royal Hospital. He was married twice; first to Elizabeth Whittle on 8 December 1651, with whom he had ten children, seven sons and three daughters. Elizabeth died on 11 August 1696. His married his second wife, Christina Hope, on 11 July 1703, with whom he had a further four children, two daughters and two sons.

As a public servant he was highly respected; remembering that this was a time when people in such high office, were prone to corruption, he was one of those who discharged their duties with an unquestionable probity.

Chapter 5

Individuals and Surgeons connected with the Hospital

William Hiseland's story is a truly remarkable one. His surname has sometimes been spelt as Hasland or even Hadeland, but to keep it simple we will refer to him as Hiseland.

As far as we know his date of birth was 6 August 1620 and he was a soldier with both the English and British armies. He died at the reputed age of 111 on 7 February 1732. He became a soldier in 1633 at the age of 13 and went on to fight at the Battle of Edgehill, in Warwickshire with King Charles I and his

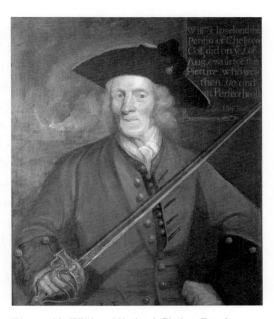

Figure 10: William Hiseland Chelsea Pensioner.

Royalist Army, on Sunday, 23 October 1642, which was the first pitched battle of the First English Civil War. At the end of the day there was no decisive victory for either side in a war that would continue for another four years.

William also fought in the Williamite War in Ireland, which took place between 12 March and 3 October 1689, when he was nearly 70 years of age.

On 11 September 1709 a battle took place near to the hamlet of Malplaquet, in the Nord region of France, during the War of the Spanish Succession. The armies of the Grand Alliance, including soldiers from Britain, the Holy Roman Empire, Austria, the United Provinces – today known as Holland – and the Danish Auxiliary Corps, under the command of the Duke of Marlborough and Prince Eugene of Savoy, were up against the French Army, led by Claude de Villars and Louis Boufflers. Even though the Grand Alliance suffered some 24,000 casualties against France's 12,500, by the rules of warfare at the time, it was the armies of the Grand Alliance who were deemed to be the victors, as it was the French Army who had retreated from the battlefield in good order, only because Boufflers, realising the battle could not be won, ordered his men to retire. This resulted in a classic pyrrhic victory for the Duke of Marlborough.

One of the men who formed part of the Grand Alliance army that day was William Hiseland of the Royal Scots. It is believed that he was 89 years of age at the time, and by far the oldest man on the battlefield. Remarkably, Hiseland had not only taken part in the English Civil Wars some seventy years earlier, but he went on to live long enough to become the last survivor from those days.

By the time his military career finally came to an end, he had reached the rank of sergeant. In recognition of his eighty years of military service, at the age of 93, he was provided with a pension of one crown a week, which was about five shillings, by the 1st Duke of Richmond, Charles Lennox, who also held the titles of 1st Duke of Lennox, as well as the 1st Duke of Aubigny. Besides being a nobleman and a politician, he was also the illegitimate son of King Charles II and his mistress, Louise de Kérouaille, the Duchess of Portsmouth. The one crown per week of Charles Lennox, was matched by Sir Robert Walpole, who went on to become the first Prime Minister of Great Britain on 4 April 1721, a position he would hold for nearly twenty-one years.

Wiliam became an in-pensioner at the Royal Hospital Chelsea, in about 1713, a place which he subsequently had to relinquish when he married ten years later at the age of 103. When his wife died, William returned as an in-pensioner at the hospital, where he remained until his death at the claimed age of 111. On his death he was buried in the hospital's small cemetery, which is situated just outside the Margaret Thatcher Infirmary wing.

The well-known painter of the day, George Alsop, painted a portrait of William Hiseland, which he sat for on 1 August 1730. The painting still exists and can be found in the Royal Hospital's museum.

George Barret (Senior) was born in Dublin around 1730 and went on to become one of Ireland's best-known landscape artists, who excelled at both water colours as well as oil paintings, although it was the latter that he was best known for. His first job though wasn't painting; in fact, it couldn't have been any further away from what he was destined to eventually do. He became an apprentice to a stay maker, which in layman's terms meant that he helped to make corsets.

George married a local girl, Frances Percy, in Dublin in 1757. Four of their children, James, George, Joseph and Mary, all went on to become painters. George junior became a member of the Society of Painters in water colours and achieved a suitable level of recognition for his artistic works. James actually succeeded his father as the master painter at the Royal Hospital Chelsea.

After finishing his studies at the Royal Dublin Society, he initially had a job teaching students how to draw. In 1762, aged 32, he took the decision to leave his beloved Ireland to find out if the streets of London really were paved with gold, and to see if he could establish himself as an artist in the city. He succeeded rather more quickly than he could have possibly expected and rapidly gained a reputation as one of the leading artists of his time.

The Society of Artists of Great Britain was formed in London in May 1761 by a group of artists who wanted to find a venue for living artists to display their works. Some of the leading artists from this society subsequently left in 1768 and formed the Royal Academy of Arts. As a result of exhibiting his works at the society, Barret was able to obtain patronage from many of the country's leading art collectors of the time. He was also one of those members who left the society to set up the Royal Academy of Art in 1768.

Barret travelled widely throughout Great Britain to paint numerous landscapes commissioned by wealthy patrons, which earned him considerable sums of money, with which he sadly wasn't good at managing. In 1782, when he was 52 years of age, he was helped by a friend of his, Edmund Burke, who was also from Dublin. He wasn't a fellow artist, but a Member of Parliament, an author, orator, political theorist and philosopher. In short, he was a man of influence.

It was on Burke's recommendation that Barret acquired the position at the Royal Hospital Chelsea, of master painter, a position he held until his death in 1784. Even though he had made large sums of money from his paintings over the years, at the time of his death his widow and children were left destitute. Thankfully for them the Royal Academy stepped in and granted Barret's widow a pension of £30 a year.

George Barret senior died on 29 May 1784 in Paddington, London, but his son James helped keep the family name respected in the art world, by exhibiting both oils and watercolours at the Royal Academy between 1785 and 1819. In 2005, a painting by George Barret, *Wooded Landscape with Fishermen Hauling in their Nets*, sold at Christies in London, for £512,000.

Whilst on the subject of paintings and artists, it would be an appropriate time to mention the painting commissioned by the Duke of Wellington in 1816. It depicted Chelsea Pensioners, drinking in the street outside the Duke of York public house across the road from the Royal Hospital Chelsea, whilst reading about Wellington's victory over Napoleon at the Battle of Waterloo in the *London Gazette*'s edition dated 22 June 1815. This had just been delivered by a cavalryman from the Marquess of Anglesey's Lancers. The painting, by the Scottish artist Sir David Wilkie, wasn't completed until 1822 and was then exhibited at the Royal Academy in London, proving to be extremely popular with the general public, maybe because of their affinity with wounded veterans.

Sir David Wilkie completed numerous sketches which he sent to Wellington to develop the Duke's original idea on what he wanted the finished painting to look like. One of the early versions of this, completed in oils, is displayed at the Royal Hospital Chelsea, although it has fewer figures than the finished painting, which Wellington paid 1200 guineas for.

A really interesting character connected to the Hospital was **Admiral John Henry Godfrey**, who was born at Handsworth in the West Midlands in July 1888, and who served in both the First and Second World Wars. His connection to the Royal Hospital came as he was the chairman of the hospital's management committee between 1949 and 1960.

It isn't his obvious connection to the hospital that makes him an interesting character, but that Ian Fleming, the author of the James Bond stories, and who worked under Godfrey in Naval Intelligence during the Second World War, based the fictional character 'M' on Godfrey, who would later somewhat whimsically complain that Fleming 'turned me into that unsavoury character M.'

Another man worth mentioning is **Sir Hew Dalrymple Ross**. Born in Scotland on 5 July 1779, he had a distinguished military career stretching from 1795 to 1858, having been educated at the Royal Military Academy, Woolwich. On 1 January 1868, he was promoted to the rank of field marshal, on 3 August 1868, he became the Lieutenant Governor of the Royal Hospital Chelsea, but just four months later, on 10 December 1868, he died at his home in Knightsbridge, London. His son was General Sir John Ross who fought in the Crimean War as well as the Indian Mutiny of 1857–1858.

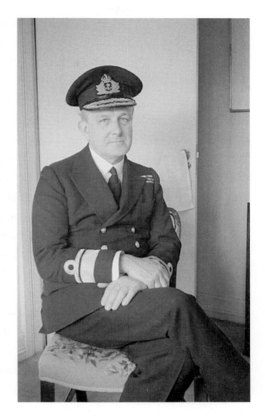

Figure 11: Admiral John Henry Godfrey, CBE.

George Robert Gleig was an extremely interesting character. He was born in Stirling, Scotland on 20 April 1796, his parents being the Bishop of Brechin and Janet Hamilton. George was educated at Stirling Grammar School. He had a scholarship to Balliol College, Oxford as a student of divinity, but in July 1813 he gave it up to join the Duke of Wellington's army, as a junior officer in the 85th Light Infantry. On 7 October that same year Wellington crossed into France from Spain for the first time and on 10 April 1814 he defeated Napoleon in what turned out to be the final battle of the Peninsular War at Toulouse. He did not find out until two days later that Napoleon had already abdicated as Emperor of France on 6 April.

Some British troops were then sent to America during the War of 1812, which lasted until 1815. There Gleig took part in five battles, at Bladensburg,

Baltimore, New Orleans, Washington and Fort Bayo, and was wounded on three occasions, but thankfully for him, not seriously. When the war ended he returned to England and continued with his scholarship, but this time at Magdalen College, Oxford, in 1816.

Whilst studying at university he married Sarah Cameron, the daughter of Captain Cameron the Younger, from Kinlochleven. Following in his father's footsteps, he took holy orders, and in 1820 became the curate of Westwell, in Kent, as well as the villages of Ash and Ivychurch. Despite being the curate to three parishes, he still found time to write a series of articles for *Blackwoods Magazine*, that had been founded by publisher, William Blackwood, in 1817. The articles were about his Peninsular War experiences, which at the time might have appeared somewhat strange to hear a man of the cloth talking about killing and war. A book was made of them in 1825, entitled *The Subaltern*. He followed this up by writing about his war time experiences in America.

Unbeknown to Gleig, he had come to the attention of the Duke of Wellington, whom he was invited to meet. He did so and went on to become a regular visitor to Wellington's home. One of the other books which Gleig wrote, was, *The Life of the Duke of Wellington*.

He was the author of some forty-nine books, three of which were about the Royal Hospital Chelsea. In 1829 he had a book published in three volumes entitled, *The Chelsea Pensioners*. This was followed in 1838 by a further two books, *Chelsea Hospital and its Traditions*, which was published in three volumes, and *The Veterans of Chelsea Hospital*, also in three volumes.

By 1832 whilst the Chaplain at the Royal Hospital Chelsea, he publicly opposed the Reform Bill that was before Parliament. Its official title was 'The Representation of the People's Act 1832', which introduced some wide-ranging changes to the electoral system throughout England and Wales. In essence the Act was intended to prevent some of the time-honoured abuses of the nation's voting system which allowed a minority powerful elite to control and dictate the balance of power in elections, with the criteria used as to who was eligible to vote differing greatly from borough to borough. The other major effect of the Act, was the massive increase in the number of people who were eligible to vote, another 300,000, which meant that about one in five adult males were enfranchised. This greatly reduced the power of the smaller wealthy elite who, prior to the new Act of Parliament, had held great power over the poorer majority of society, a status quo that they wanted to keep.

Ultimately the Bill failed, but only by forty-one votes, and the masses were not happy at all. Riots and violence ensued, breaking out the very evening of the failure of the Bill. Bristol saw the worst of it, where the Palace of the Bishop of Bristol was destroyed along with the mansion of the Lord Mayor. The prison was broken into and inmates were released, whilst in several cities buildings were destroyed along with private homes.

Despite voting against the Bill, Gleig fell out with the Duke of Wellington, with whom he had previously been on very good terms, when in 1840, he announced that he intended to begin educating non-commissioned officers as well as private soldiers. The duke was outraged at Gleig's announcement of his intentions, so much so that he publicly reprimanded him. Wellington did not see the need for men from the other ranks to be educated. They simply had to do what they were told to do by their officers, that was it, plain and simple. They did not require independent thought to do what they needed to do in battle. Wellington said of the matter: '*By Jove! If there is mutiny in the army, and in all probability we shall have one, you'll see that these new fangled schoolmasters will be at the bottom of it.*'

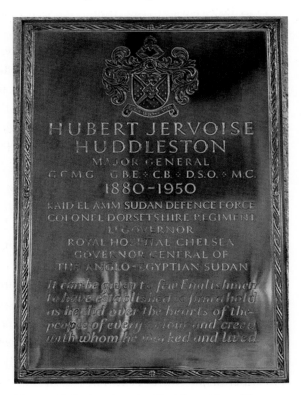

Figure 12: Hubert Jervoise Huddleton Brass Plaque (Creative Commons International Licence).

Until that point in time the upper classes and the aristocracy had had it all their own way and were in no mood to give up the power that had been in their hands and that of their families for generations.

Despite his very public disagreement with the Duke of Wellington, Gleig was appointed the Chaplain General of the Armed Forces in 1844, a post he held for the next thirty-one years before he resigned, by which time he was 79 years of age. During that same time he was also the Inspector General of Military Schools. Gleig died in Hampshire in 1888.

Major General Sir Hubert Jervoise Huddleston GCMG GBE CB DSO & Bar MC was born on 20 January 1880 and served in the British Army for 49 years between 1898 and 1947. In 1900 he was commissioned from the ranks of the Coldstream Guards for valour in the Second Boer War and later served with the Dorsetshire Regiment where he was Mentioned in Despatches twice and saw action in the Orange Free State and the Transvaal in 1900, including the Battle of Diamond Hill.

He also served during the First World War and was a key figure in the Dafur Campaign of 1916 where he commanded an Australian battalion in the Imperial Camel Corps and was awarded the DSO twice. He commanded a brigade throughout General Allenby's Palestine Campaign of 1917–18. He remained in the Army after the war and was promoted to General Officer Commanding Sudan in 1924. In 1930 he was placed in command of the British Army's 14th Infantry Brigade. Between 1934 and 1938, he was stationed at different postings in India. He was Commander of the Eastern Command in 1934 and the following year he was given the same position, but in charge of the Western Command. His wartime awards included the Distinguished Service Order and Bar, along with the Military Cross.

In early 1940 he was appointed Lieutenant Governor and Secretary of the Royal Hospital Chelsea, but this turned out to be extremely short term, as in April that year he was appointed General Officer Commanding Northern Ireland. This was just as short a posting as when he was at the Royal Hospital, as he only remained in Ireland until July that year, before being appointed Governor General of Anglo-Egyptian Sudan, later that year, a position that he retained until 1947 when he retired from the British Army.

Over the years there were some very eminent surgeons who worked at the Royal Hospital Chelsea. The issue of surgeons, how they came into being as a professional and officially recognised body, and how they were connected to barbers, is a story in itself which is covered in more detail towards the end of this chapter. Below are some of the surgeons who worked at the Royal Hospital Chelsea over the years. Not all are mentioned but those that are represent all of those who served the hospital so splendidly over the years.

Messenger Monsey was born in October 1694 in the sleepy hollow of Hackford-with-Whitwell in Norfolk. His education saw him a student at the prestigious Pembroke College, Cambridge, where he was awarded a BA in 1714, before deciding to study medicine. He studied and worked hard and in 1723 he was admitted to the Royal College of Physicians.

Monsey's real break came when he was called to attend to Francis Godolphin, 2nd Earl of Godolphin who had been taken ill with what was then termed as apoplexy, but what is today more commonly known as a stroke. Godolphin was immediately taken by Monsey's undoubted skill as a physician, his outlandish sense of humour and what he saw as Monsey's insolent, border-line rude, familiarity. Godolphin pushed the matter further and managed to convince Monsey that he should move to London. It was the right decision,

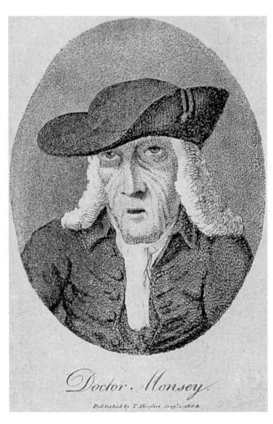

Figure 13: Messenger Monsey (Creative Commons International Licence).

as Godolphin introduced him to his celebrity friends, who included the then Prime Minister, Sir Robert Walpole, and Lord Chesterfield, who was a British statesman, diplomat, a literary man, as well as being an accomplished wit.

Monsey's personality didn't suit everyone. His frankness and directness, were not always appreciated in the circles in which he now found himself. Some of these individuals, although rich, powerful and influential, were quite fragile creatures underneath the surface, who liked their egos to be massaged by those around them, and certainly did not always like to hear the truth, let alone be told it face to face by somebody who they perhaps saw as beneath them in the social pecking order. One such individual Monsey fell out with was the distinguished eighteenth-century actor and playwright, David Garrick.

The eighteenth-century writer, poet, biographer and literary critic, Samuel Johnson, who was often referred to as Dr Johnson, greatly disapproved of what he described as Monsey's coarse wit, whilst the diarist Fanny Burney, described him as 'Dr Monso' and being 'a strange gross man'.

As Monsey grew older, so his bluntness, profanities and vulgar language increased in its usage. William Munk, a physician and also a member of the Royal College of Physicians, but one who was born some 30 years after Monsey died, described him in these words:

Monsey maintained his original plainness of manners, and with an unreserved sincerity sometimes spoke truth in a manner that gave offence; and as old age approached, he acquired an asperity of behaviour and a neglect of decorum.

Monsey acquired his position at the Royal Hospital Chelsea, which also came with accommodation in apartments located in part of the old college, via his connection to Francis Godolphin and, despite the fact he despised modern improvements in theory and practice, he kept his job there until his death at the hospital on Boxing Day 1788, when he was 96 years of age.

On his death he left £16,000 to his daughter and only child, Charlotte, and he bequeathed his body to medical science in keeping with his wishes. He was dissected in a post mortem examination in front of medical students at Guy's Hospital, soon after his death.

John Ranby was born in 1703, the son of Joseph Ranby, an inn keeper of St Giles-in-the-Fields, Middlesex. Where young John Ranby's desire to become involved in surgery, came from is not recorded. But on 5 April 1715, at the tender age of just 12 years, he became an apprentice to Edward Barnard, who was a foreign brother of the Company of Barber-Surgeons.

Barber-Surgeons, who were one of the most common medical practitioners, had been about since the Middle Ages, which in historical terms refers to the one thousand year period between the fifth and fifteenth centuries, although the first mention of the Company of Barber-Surgeons dates back to 1308, when a Richard Barbour, was elected by the Court of Aldermen, to keep order amongst his fellow barbers. Their main purpose had been to tend to the wounds of soldiers during or after a battle. Barber surgeons had been around a long time and had been working in monasteries since around 1,000 AD. The reason for this, was because before the founding of the Royal Hospital Chelsea, old soldiers had historically been looked after and treated by monks in their monasteries. But the monks were forbidden to 'spill blood' so they had to employ barber surgeons to do this for them.

In 1540 an Act of Parliament had amalgamated the Surgeons Guild and the Company of Barbers, which amongst its advantages, provided the new company with the right to the bodies of four executed criminals for dissection each year. The Act separated the different functions of barbers and surgeons and they were not allowed to undertake each other's work. Surgeons were not permitted to cut hair or shave other men, whilst barbers were forbidden to practise surgery, other than to extract teeth. In fact, the old fashioned red and white barber's pole which hung outside a hairdresser's, or a barber's shop as it was called when I was a boy, represented the two crafts. Red for surgery and white for barbering.

Barber's received higher wages than surgeons until surgeons were entered into British warships during naval wars. With the rising professionalism of surgery, in 1745 surgeons officially broke away from barbers to form the company of surgeons, which in 1800, became the Royal College of Surgeons.

During those years, what is today referred to as surgery, was usually carried out by barbers and not physicians. Barbers throughout Europe would carry out a wide spectrum of tasks ranging from blood letting, the pulling of teeth, cutting hair, neck manipulation, cleansing of ears and scalp, lancing of boils, ulcers and cysts, enemas and the amputation of limbs. Understandably, the survival rates of post surgical procedures, was generally quite low mainly due to the loss of blood and infection.

Surprising as it might seem to us today, physicians considered surgery to be beneath them. They tended to come from wealthy and powerful families and were academics and theologians, who worked in universities and saw their role when it came to working with the sick, as that of an observer, or a consultant. They appear literally to have not wanted to get their hands dirty.

To return to John Ranby, after having been an apprentice for some seven years, and still only 19 years of age, he was given the seal of the Barber Surgeons Company as a foreign brother on 5 October 1722, after he had passed an examination on his skill in surgery. Just two years later, and still only 21 years of age, he was elected as a fellow of the Royal Society on 30 November 1724.

His reputation as a skilled surgeon made him a sought after by the rich and famous of the day at such times as when they required surgery. Such was his notoriety that in 1738 he was appointed surgeon-in-ordinary to the Royal household. After just two years of serving the Royal family he was promoted to the position of sergeant-surgeon to King George II, and in May 1743 he became the principal sergeant-surgeon to the king.

King George embarked on a campaign in what is now Germany later in the year of 1743. As his personal surgeon, John Ranby accompanied him and was present at the Battle of Dettingen. There he treated Prince William, Duke of Cumberland, who was one of the king's sons. He received a musket ball wound to one of his legs. Fortunately, Ranby was able to remove the offending shot without causing too much damage or without having to resort to amputating the wounded leg.

He was appointed as surgeon to the Royal Hospital Chelsea on 13 May 1752 and held the position for 21 years up to the time of his death on 28 August 1773.

Ranby had been described as a man of strong passions, with a harsh voice, and inelegant manners. Queen Caroline of Ansbach referred to him as 'the blockhead' but still allowed him to operate on her in relation to an umbilical hernia on 9 November 1737. She took to her bed and during the next few days she was operated on by Ranby without anaesthetic. On 17 November her strangulated bowel burst, and she died three days later on 20 November 1737 at St James's Palace, London. She had originally suffered the hernia at the birth of her last child in 1724.

Messenger Monsey, who as described above in the previous entry, wasn't exactly the most liked man of his day, didn't particularly hold him in high esteem. Monsey was reported to have said: '*Ranby was the only man I ever heard coolly defend the use of laudanum in effecting his designs on women, which he had practised with success.*'

Ranby wrote the following works.

- Three curious Dissections by John Ranby, esq., Surgeon to His Majesty's Household and Fellow of Royal Surgeons *(1728)*.
- The Method of Treating Gunshot Wounds *(1744)*.
- A Narrative of the last illness of Earl of Orford, from May 1744 to the day of his decease, 18 March following *(1745)*.
- The true account of all the Transactions before the Right Honourable the Lords and others, Commissioners for the affairs of Chelsea Hospital as far as it relates to the Admission and Dismission of Samuel Lee, Surgeon *(1754)*.

Other Surgeons

John Noades began working at the hospital on 18 August 1690. He died in 1752 and was buried in the grounds of the Royal Hospital Chelsea.

Alex Inglis started life at the Royal Hospital on 16 March 1706 and died on 26 January 1736. He is buried in the Royal Hospital Chelsea's burial ground.

Sir Thomas Renton became the hospital's surgeon on 3 February 1721 and died on 30 November 1740. He was buried in the hospital's burial ground.

William Chesleden started working at the hospital on 27 January 1736. He was a well-respected anatomist and had some of his works published, including, *The Anatomy of the Human Body*. He has been written about in more detail elsewhere in this book.

Robert Adair began working at the Royal Hospital Chelsea on 1 September 1773. He later became the Surgeon General of the Army in 1783 and was also Sergeant Surgeon to King George III.

Thomas Keate was the chief surgeon at the Royal Hospital Chelsea from 17 March 1790, and is one of those buried in the hospital's grounds. He was also the Master of the Royal College of Surgeons on three occasions, in 1802, 1809, and 1818.

Sir Everard Home began his stint as the chief surgeon at the Royal Hospital Chelsea on 25 July 1821. He was also a lecturer on anatomy, as well as the first President of the Royal College of Surgeons. After his death on 31 August 1832, the posts of Surgeon and Physician at the Royal Hospital, were combined.

Everard Home gained a scholarship to Trinity College, Cambridge, but despite this, he trained under his brother-in-law, John Hunter at St George's Hospital, which was, and still is a teaching hospital in Tooting, London.

He was appointed as the assistant surgeon at Plymouth Naval Hospital in 1778. He later became the assistant surgeon, and surgeon at St George's Hospital, and in 1808 he became the Sergeant Surgeon to King George III.

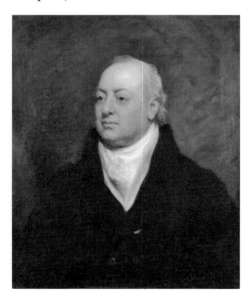

Figure 14: Sir Everard Home.

Physicians & Surgeons

Daniel McLachlin began working at the Royal Hospital Chelsea on 8 May 1840.

William Lucas was the Principal Medical Officer at the Royal Hospital Chelsea, a position he began on 1 July 1863.

John Alex McMunn was appointed as the physician and surgeon at the Royal Hospital Chelsea on 4 November 1868. Prior to this, Mr McMunn had also been the Hospital's Deputy Surgeon, a position he began on 11 November 1862.

Thomas Ligertwood became the surgeon at the Royal Hospital Chelsea on 3 June 1896, holding the rank of colonel, finally retiring from the Army on 3 June 1904. He had served with the Royal Army Medical Corps during the Crimean War 1854–56, where he saw action at the Battle of Alma, for which he was Mentioned in Despatches and at the Battle of Inkerman, where he was slightly wounded, the capture of Balaklava and the assault on the Redan in June 1955.

He died, still in post, on 10 May 1911 at the age of 81 and was buried in the grounds of the hospital. Prior to his appointment as the surgeon, he had also held the position of deputy surgeon at the hospital, having commenced that role on 13 January 1869.

Charles Seymour MB began in the position as surgeon of the Royal Hospital Chelsea on 3 June 1904, when he was a lieutenant colonel in the Royal Army Medical Corps. He retired from the position on 31 December 1909.

Reginald James Cope Cottell first qualified as a doctor in 1885 having studied at St George's Training Hospital in London, after deciding to follow his brother into the world of medicine. Within just a few years he joined the Royal Army Medical Corps as a probationary surgeon. In 1906 he was appointed as a junior assistant surgeon at the Royal Hospital Chelsea, succeeding to the senior post of physician and surgeon on 1 January 1910, whilst serving as a lieutenant colonel with the Royal Army Medical Corps. He continued in the top position until he retired in 1913.

Whilst working at the Royal Hospital he carried out some excellent work, both medically and surgically, in caring for the in-pensioners' health and seeing that their infirmities were treated by the most up to date methods, both operatively and by non-invasive means. He also involved himself in the hospital's work in relation to Army pensions in a time before there was a Ministry of Pensions.

The beginning of the First World War brought him out of his military retirement to undertake recruitment duties for the British Government. In 1915 his medical skills were once again needed, when he was put in command of King George's Hospital, a Red Cross Hospital situated in the premises of His Majesty's Stationary Office in Stamford Street, Waterloo Bridge Road.

Sir Oliver Richard Archer Julian CB was appointed surgeon of the Royal Hospital on 13 October 1913. He was a lieutenant colonel in the Royal Army Medical Corps and left his coveted position on 23 June 1915 for active service in France, where he arrived on 14 July.

He was awarded the Victory Medal, British War Medal, 15 Star as well as the General Service Medal for his wartime military service. His First World War British Army Medal Rolls index card shows two postwar addresses for him, one being Balfour House, Finsbury Pavement, London, and the other c/o, Messrs Holt and Co, 3 Whitehall Hall Place, London, SW1. Holt and Co were London bankers who started out as Army Agents, providing current accounts for many officers of the British Army.

Lieutenant Colonel George Arthur Theodore Bray DSO became the physician and surgeon at the Royal Hospital Chelsea on 24 June 1914. He served with the Royal Army Medical Corps and had previously been the deputy surgeon at the Royal Hospital, a role he had commenced on 20 January 1914. He was another who left his position of comparative safety at the Royal Hospital in affluent Chelsea, and went active service, first arriving in France on 19 November 1915. For his wartime service, he was awarded the 1915 Star, the British War Medal and the British Victory Medal. His postwar address was shown in the First World War Army medal index as 10 Miles Road, Clifton, Bristol.

Sir Augustus Alexander Brooke-Pechell was a retired lieutenant colonel who had served with the Royal Army Medical Corps. He was another who had previously been a deputy surgeon working at the hospital, a role he had begun on 24 June 1915, resigning his position on 30 April 1919. He died on 6 October 1937, two months after his 80th birthday.

Major Frederick E. Roberts DSO took up the role of physician and surgeon on June 1919, but his appointment was always intended to be temporary, until a full-time replacement could be found to replace Sir Augustus.

Major Richard James Campbell Thompson CMG, DSO arrived in France on 22 August 1914, just a matter of days in to the war as part of the British Expeditionary Force. At the time he held the rank of captain in the Royal Army Medical Corps. He was awarded the 14 Star, the British War Medal as well as the Victory Medal, for his wartime military service. His Army medal rolls index card, shows he eventually reached the rank of lieutenant colonel and that his medals were sent to the Royal Hospital Chelsea. He became the physician surgeon at the Royal Hospital Chelsea on 23 July 1919, a position he held for three years before retiring on 23 July 1922.

Major Edmund Thurlow Potts CMG DSO MiD is shown as serving in South Africa at the time of the 1911 Census, at which time he was a captain in the Royal Army Medical Corps. He became the physician surgeon at the Royal Hospital Chelsea on 24 July 1922.

Assistant Surgeons

William North began working as an assistant surgeon at the Royal Hospital Chelsea, on 15 June 1809. He died on 23 November 1816 aged 72, and was buried at Old Cemetery, Kings Road, London.

John Hartshorn took up his position as assistant surgeon at the Royal Hospital Chelsea on 31 July 1816. On the death of Mr Leeds, the deputy surgeon, who died on 24 November 1829, Mr Hartshorn was promoted to that office, and that of assistant surgeon was abolished until the year 1846.

Alexander Adam Prout took up the position of assistant surgeon at the Royal Hospital Chelsea on 8 September 1846. He died in October 1854.

Francis Holton was appointed as an assistant surgeon at the Royal Hospital Chelsea on 10 February 1857.

Arthur H.F. Taylor took up his appointment as the assistant surgeon at the Royal Hospital Chelsea on 22 November 1858.

Howison Young Howison was appointed as an assistant surgeon on 21 August 1859. On 1 July 1863 Mr Howison was transferred to work at the Royal Military Asylum, which was a school and a home for the children of fallen soldiers.

Deputy Surgeons

John E. Leeds became the deputy surgeon at the Royal Hospital Chelsea, on 15 June 1809.

Thomas Coke Gaulter became the deputy surgeon at the Royal Hospital Chelsea on 8 September 1846.

W.J. MacNamara MiD, became the deputy surgeon at the Royal Hospital Chelsea on 4 August 1896. He was a surgeon major in the Royal Army Medical Corps. He served in the British Army during the First World War at which time he held the rank of lieutenant colonel and during his time serving in France, he was Mentioned in Despatches. He retired from the Royal Hospital on the completion of his term of appointment.

Richard William Ford DSO was appointed as deputy surgeon at the Royal Hospital Chelsea on 17 August 1901. He was a lieutenant colonel in the Royal Army Medical Corps and resigned after having completed his agreed term of office on 16 August 1906.

Major Francis Kiddle MB began his appointment as the deputy surgeon at the Royal Hospital Chelsea on 1 January 1910 whilst serving in the Royal Army Medical Corps but resigned his appointment prior to the completion of his term of office. This was possibly due to the outbreak of the war as records show that he arrived in France on 15 August 1914 as part of the British Expeditionary Force, just eleven days after the outbreak of hostilities. By the end of the war he had been promoted to the rank of lieutenant colonel and awarded the 1914 Star along with the British War and Victory Medals for his wartime military service. His address at the time of applying for his medals was shown as Brooke House, Francis Street, London WC1.

Major Herbert E. Winter began his appointment as the deputy surgeon of the Royal Hospital Chelsea 1 March 1912. He served in the Royal Army Medical Corps, having transferred from the Foreign Service.

Captain H.G. Coulthard was appointed as a deputy surgeon at the Royal Hospital Chelsea on 17 November 1915, but subsequently transferred to an un-named Queen Alexandra's Military Hospital on 13 May 1918. He was a captain in the Royal Army Medical Corps.

Captain T.H.F. Roberts was appointed to the position of deputy surgeon at the Royal Hospital Chelsea on 14 May 1918. He left and returned to civilian life on being demobilized from the Royal Army Medical Corps, on 12 May 1919.

This incredible group of men had all served their country in a military role, which provided them with an understanding and a level of empathy that was required to properly oversee the needs and welfare of the veterans of the Royal Hospital Chelsea, an understanding that was the minimum that they deserved.

Chapter 6

Margaret Thatcher

Margaret Thatcher, or the Iron Lady, as she was famously dubbed in 1976 by Captain Yuri Gavrilov of the then Soviet Union Army, was born Margaret Hilda Roberts on 13 October 1925 at Grantham in Lincolnshire, the younger daughter of Alfred and Beatrice Roberts. Home was a flat above one of the two grocery shops that her father owned, who was an astute and clever man. He was a local alderman who was quite high up in Lincolnshire County Council, a God-fearing man who was also a local preacher, and he was the Mayor of Grantham between November 1945 and November 1946.

As a young girl Margaret would listen to Churchill's wartime speeches on the wireless, which was one of the reasons for her mistrust of the Germans, a feeling which stayed with her into her adult years. This lack of trust was endorsed when a young Austrian Jewish girl called Edith, came to stay with them for a while. She explained in great detail how Hitler and his Nazi party had persecuted the Jews in Austria after they had invaded and occupied the country in 1938. Margaret never forgot the stories that

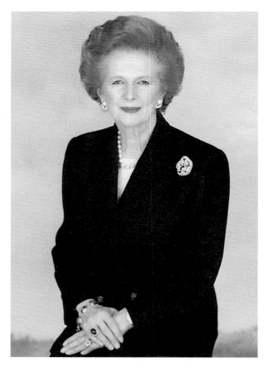

Figure 15: The Rt. Hon. Margaret Thatcher.

Edith had told her, and nowhere was this better highlighted than at the time of the fall of the Berlin Wall and the re-unification of Germany. Whilst the rest of the world rejoiced at a divided nation once again becoming a single entity, after a period of 44 years, Margaret Thatcher's concern was that a united Germany would revert to type and once again seek world domination. This was a country that she never truly trusted.

In her school days she excelled academically and went on to become the head girl; she was in every sense a model student. She also took a keen interest in reading, poetry, hockey, swimming and walking.

Her parents were not particularly wealthy so she successfully applied for a scholarship to study Chemistry at Somerville College, Oxford, which was founded in 1879 and named after the Scottish scientist and mathematician, Mary Somerville, to allow those who would have otherwise been excluded from such an education, to be included.

She met her husband, Dennis Thatcher, who was a successful businessman, at a dinner to celebrate her formal adoption as the Conservative Party candidate for Dartford in the 1951 General Election. She was subsequently defeated by the Labour candidate, Norman Dodds, who had also previously defeated her in the General Election of the previous year. She had moved to Dartford around that time and worked as a research chemist for J. Lyons & Co.

Her mainstream political career began in 1959 when she was elected as the Conservative Member of Parliament for Finchley. During Edward Heath's time as Prime Minister, between 1970 and 1974, she was made Secretary of State for Education and Science, before becoming leader of the Conservative Party on 11 February 1975 and Prime Minister on 4 May 1979, the first time in British history a woman had held such high office, a position she held until 28 November 1990.

Margaret, by then, Baroness Thatcher, died on 8 April 2013 after suffering a stroke and was given a ceremonial funeral with full military honours at St Paul's Cathedral in London, nine days after her death.

A service took place on 28 September 2013 in All Saints Chapel at the Royal Hospital's Margaret Thatcher Infirmary, which bears her name and which was opened by her and His Royal Highness, Prince Charles, in 2009.

After the service her ashes were interred in the hospital's burial ground, immediately outside the Infirmary, next to those of her husband, Dennis Thatcher, whose ashes were similarly laid to rest there in a ceremony on 3 July 2003, after his death on 26 June 2003.

Margaret Thatcher had been a long-standing supporter as well as a neighbour of the Royal Hospital Chelsea for many years, a place that she visited on a regular basis, and where she also regularly attended church services in the hospital's chapel. There is a bust and a portrait of her at the hospital, both of which can be found in the Margaret Thatcher Infirmary, which can hold up to 100 patients at any one time. It is a five-star care home which provides quality nursing for the hospitals' elderly residents, along with therapists. The building also includes a gymnasium and a hydrotherapy pool, as well as numerous activities for the pensioners to take advantage of, offering both physical exercise and mental stimulation.

The 2016 annual report of the Care Quality Commission, an independent regulator of health and social care throughout England, marked the Margaret Thatcher Infirmary at the Royal Hospital Chelsea in the following five categories.

SAFE: Good

This meant that qualified nursing staff administered and recorded which medicines, each patient received, when and how often. The Royal Hospital ensured that there were sufficient staffing levels on duty at all times to cater for the number of patients who required treatment. There were risk assessments in place to identify potential areas of risk, and to reduce the possibility of any patient coming to harm. The training that each of the staff received was refreshed on an annual basis

EFFECTIVE: Good

The infirmary's staff were aware of each patient's medical status and responded quickly to deal with any changing conditions which may have arisen to individual patients, who had access to a doctor, occupational therapists, physiotherapists, as well as speech and language therapists.

Patients received appropriate care, based on their personal needs and requirements, which included a balanced diet which catered for what they wanted, whilst taking into account their medical needs. All staff were passionate about their work and understood their individual responsibilities under the Medical Capacity Act 2005 and the Deprivation of Liberty Safeguards.

CARING: Outstanding

The service provided by staff under this heading was classed as being outstanding. Staff were observed whilst treating their patients with respect and kindness and promoting their independence and dignity. Patients, and their relatives where applicable, were kept informed about their health and well-being and were kept actively involved in such decisions which directly affected them. Patients commented on how incredibly kind and compassionate staff were towards them, which in turn had a positive impact on their lives. Each patient has a designated member of staff whom they meet with on a weekly basis. When a patient has reached what is called, end of life care, they and their families are fully supported by the staff, at a time that is extremely emotional and traumatic for all concerned.

RESPONSIVE: Outstanding

Patients had a wide variety of trips, events and activities which were available to them. This including a well-equipped gymnasium, a licenced bar, a chapel for prayer and contemplation and a well-situated coffee shop. Detailed and personalised records were kept for each patient so that the staff were aware of their individual needs. These records were easily accessible by the staff and could be updated by them as when they needed to be, ensuring that the records were as up to date as possible. Patients and their families were encouraged to provide the staff with any and all relevant feedback about their care and treatment, which if received was expediently acted upon. The complaints procedure was straightforward and uncomplicated, and patients and their relatives said they would be comfortable doing so if they needed to.

WELL-LED: Outstanding

The service provided by the infirmary staff was deemed to be outstandingly well-led. This accolade came from the patients and their relatives. The manager of the infirmary was a dedicated individual and was often seen throughout the facility. The staff praised their own management team, whom they felt were very supportive, which allowed them to concentrate on their work in an unhindered manner. The quality of the service provided by the Royal Hospital was monitored by a number of audits and staff meetings, to highlight any concerns that may have arisen. Any that had been, were documented, discussed and acted upon expediently, to improve the lives and well-being of the infirmary's patients.

The full version of the report that I have mentioned and referred to above, is available to read or download on the Care Quality Commission's own website.

Chapter 7

The Class of 2017

I n this chapter we will look at a few of the individuals who are residents of the Royal Hospital, along with someone who worked there at the time this book was written.

The current crop of some 300 residents at the hospital, include those who have served their country during the Second World War, the Korean War, the Falklands War, Cyprus and the well-documented Troubles in Northern Ireland. Their home is in one of the wealthiest parts of London, and their back garden is one of the largest, most relaxing and picturesque it is possible to have.

Despite its salubrious beginnings the hospital now relies in part on charitable donations to cover its day to day costs. Its other main source of income is the monies it charges each resident in rent to live in the hospital.

To reiterate, to become a Chelsea Pensioner a man or a woman first has to be able to meet a set criteria, before being considered as an in-patient. They have to be over 65 years of age and have served as a regular soldier. They need to be in receipt of an Army Service Pension or a War Disability Pension, which is required to be surrendered upon entry to the Royal Hospital as a Chelsea Pensioner.

Those who had been commissioned officers during their period of military service can also apply, but before having received their commission, they must have previously served in the ranks for at least twelve years.

In April 2017 I visited the Royal Hospital Chelsea to speak with in-pensioner **Bill Speakman** in relation to a book I am writing on the Victoria Cross winners from the Korean War, of whom there were four. Two were posthumous awards, the first of which went to Major Kenneth Muir, The Argyll and Sutherland Highlanders (Princess Louise's) for his actions on 23 September 1950. The second was awarded to Lieutenant Philip Edward Curtis, of the Duke of Cornwall's Light Infantry, who was attached to The

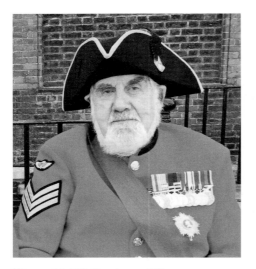

Figure 16: Bill Speakman, VC.

Gloucestershire Regiment, for his actions on 23 April 1951.

Lieutenant Colonel James Power Carne DSO, also of The Gloucestershire Regiment, and during the same actions as Lieutenant Curtis, was awarded the Victoria Cross for his bravery. He died in Cheltenham, Gloucestershire on 19 April 1986, at the age of 80. This left Bill Speakman as the only living recipient of the Victoria Cross awarded during the Korean War, as of 2017.

When I interviewed him he still cut an impressive looking figure of a man, even at 89 years of age. At 6ft 5in tall, he still had an imposing look about him. When I asked Bill about his actions in November 1951 that saw him awarded the Victoria Cross, the highest bravery award that there is in the United Kingdom's honours system for gallantry in the face of the enemy, he must have been overcome with an

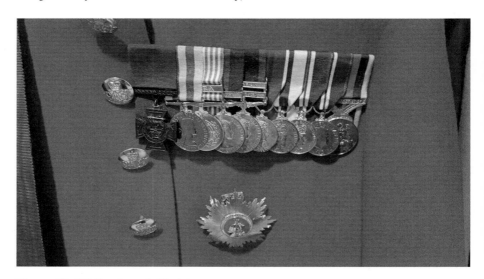

Figure 17: Bill Speakman's Medals.

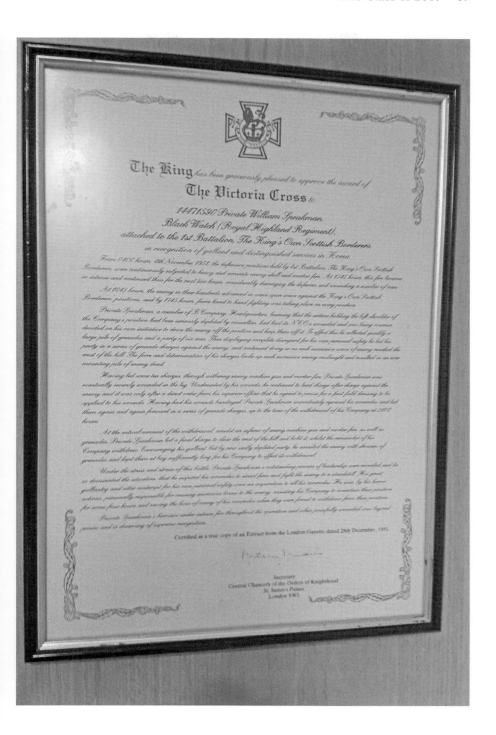

attack of modesty. His answer was: '*I was on this hill with my mates and they were trying to kill us all, and I didn't want to die. That was it really.*'

Well, that most definitely wasn't it at all. On the wall in Bill's room at the hospital is the citation for the award of his Victoria Cross. It reads as follows:

The King has been graciously pleased to approve the award of
The Victoria Cross *to:*
14471590 Private William Speakman
Black Watch (Royal Highland Regiment).
attached to the 1ˢᵗ Battalion, The King's Own Scottish Borderers
in recognition of gallant and distinguished services in Korea.

From 0400 hours 4ᵗʰ November 1951, the defensive positions held by 1ˢᵗ Battalion, The King's Own Scottish Borderers were continuously subjected to heavy and accurate enemy shell and mortar fire. At 1545 hrs., this fire became intense and continued thus for the next two hours, considerably damaging the defences and wounding a number of men.

At 1645 hrs. the enemy in their hundreds advanced in wave upon wave against the King's Own Scottish Borderers' positions, and by 1745 hrs. fierce hand-to-hand fighting was taking place on every position.

Private Speakman, a member of 'B' Company, Headquarters, learning that the section holding the left shoulder of the company's position had been seriously depleted by casualties, had had its NCO's wounded and was being over-run, decided on his own initiative to drive the enemy off the position and keep them off of it. To effect this he collected quickly a large pile of grenades and a party of six men. Then displaying complete disregard for his own personal safety, he led his party in a series of grenade charges against the enemy; and continued doing so as each successive wave of enemy reached the crest of the hill. The force and determination of his charges broke up each successive enemy onslaught and resulted in an ever-mounting pile of enemy dead.

Having led some ten charges, through withering enemy machine gun and mortar fire, Private Speakman was eventually severely wounded in the leg. Undaunted by his wounds, he continued to lead charge after charge against the enemy, and it was only after a direct order from his superior officer that he agreed to pause for a first field dressing to be applied to his wounds.

Having had his wounds bandaged, Private Speakman immediately re-joined his comrades and led them again and again forward in a series of grenade charges, up to the time of the withdrawal of his company at 2100 hrs.

At the critical moment of the withdrawal, amidst an inferno of enemy machine-gun fire and mortar fire, as well as grenades, Private Speakman led a final charge to clear the crest of the hill and hold it, whilst the remainder of his company withdrew. Encouraging his gallant but by now sadly depleted party, he assailed the enemy with showers of grenades and kept them at bay sufficiently long for his company to effect its withdrawal.

Under the stress and strain of this battle, Private Speakman's outstanding powers of leadership were revealed, and he so dominated the situation that he inspired his comrades to stand firm and fight the enemy to a standstill.

His great gallantry and utter contempt for his own personal safety were an inspiration to all his comrades. He was, by his heroic actions, personally responsible for causing enormous losses to the enemy, assisting his company to maintain their position for some four hours and saving the lives of many of his comrades when they were forced to withdraw from their position.

Private Speakman's heroism under intense fire throughout the operation and when painfully wounded was beyond praise and is deserving of supreme recognition. (London Gazette 28ᵗʰ December 1951).

After reading the above citation, you can understand what I mean by him being overcome with an attack of modesty, as these two descriptions of his actions on 4 November 1951, differ greatly.

I decided to push Bill on the matter, and although he furnished me with a bit more information, it was clear that he was not comfortable in promoting his own part on that fateful day. He went out of his way to emphasize that it wasn't just his actions that saved the day, but rather a team effort by all of his colleagues.

When Bill had seen the numbers of the enemy they were up against, literally thousands of North Koreans, he quickly realised that firing their bolt-action rifles, even if every single round counted, wasn't going to achieve much, and certainly wasn't going to stop their position from being overrun. He also worked out that the answer to their predicament was grenades, and lots of them. He and a couple of his colleagues gathered together as many grenades as they could find and started throwing them at the North Koreans as they advanced up the hill towards them. What helped Bill and his mates, was that the ground was hard, so when they threw their grenades, rather than sticking in the earth, they bounced and rolled down the hill, exploding amongst their enemy who were intent on killing them and taking their position at the top of Hill 217.

Whilst Bill was describing throwing the grenades, this is part of what he said:

> *I realised that with the ground being so hard, the only weapons we had that were going to be effective, were the grenades. Luckily for us they worked, and that was that. I didn't see what I did as being particularly brave or courageous, we all did what we had been trained to do, and that was fight. I for one certainly wasn't going to allow myself to be taken prisoner.*

I mention the above because the previous year, on 17 August 1950, on a hill above the South Korean town of Waegwan known locally as Apsan and in military terms referred to as Hill 303, was the scene of a massacre. Elements of the North Korean Army executed forty-two American prisoners who had been captured three days earlier. There were only four survivors. What made it even more of an atrocity was that all the Americans had their hands tied behind their backs and were shot from behind. So Bill's desire not to be taken prisoner by the North Koreans was a sound one.

There is no suggestion on my part that all North Korean soldiers would have acted in the same manner, but those whom Bill was up against might have reacted in the same way having had such a large number of their colleagues killed and wounded by him and his comrades.

Although Bill was awarded his Victoria Cross by King George VI, the king died on 6 February 1952, and so Bill, accompanied by his mother, was presented with his award at the first investiture undertaken by Queen Elizabeth II, at Buckingham Palace on 27 February 1952.

Bill was later promoted to the rank of sergeant and went on to serve with the Special Air Service in Malaya and Borneo, serving in the army for twenty-two years, before retiring at the age of 40 in 1967. He sold his original Victoria Cross because of financial hardship, using most of the money he received for it on a new roof for his cottage, but he was later provided with a genuine replacement by the government, which is now on display at the National War Museum of Scotland in Edinburgh. On a visit to Seoul on 21 April 2015, he presented a copy of his Victoria Cross and his other medals to the people and government of South Korea.

Bill became an in-pensioner at the Royal Hospital Chelsea 3 February 2015 but sadly passed away before this book was published on 22 June 2018.

Staff Sergeant Military Provost Staff **Jimmy Nicholson** epitomises the true character of an in-pensioner at the Royal Hospital. He is intelligent, dedicated and an extremely witty individual. But, as with all of the hospital's residents, Jimmy has his own, unique, personal story which brought him to this moment in time, this place in his life, long before he even stepped through the doors of this great British institution and it is important to include that aspect of his life as part of his story.

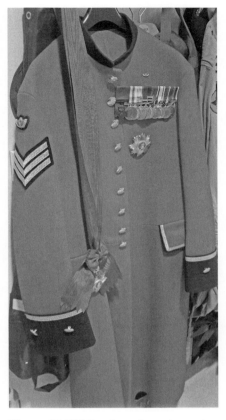

Figure 18: Bill Speakman's scarlet tunic.

We had the pleasure of meeting Jimmy in the Royal Hospital's museum, on a lovely warm spring day in April 2017. He is a very personable individual, someone to whom we immediately warmed as if we had known him for years.

Jimmy was born in Forres in the county of Moray in Scotland in 1929 and, after leaving school at the age of fifteen, he spent three years training as an undertaker. On the completion of his apprenticeship he was called up for National Service, but he chose to sign on with The Scots Guards as at the time they were offering

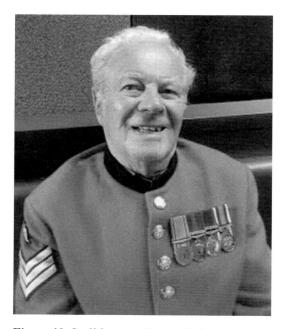

Figure 19: Staff Sergeant Jimmy Nicholson.

men who agreed to do three year's service with them, the opportunity to apply to join the Police when they had done their time.

His Army career began in October 1947, and after finishing his initial training he found himself serving in both Palestine and Egypt. During this time he became an accomplished piper.

Having completed his three years service with the Scots Guards, he applied to join the City of Aberdeen Police Force, but as Jimmy was under the strict height requirements that were in place at the time, he was not accepted. 'Very particular in those days,' were the words Jimmy used to describe his rejection. But rather than sit around feeling sorry for himself, he re-joined the Army and this time opted for the Royal Electrical & Mechanical Engineers (REME) instead. After he had undergone a course of drill instruction at the Army Training Centre at Alexander Barracks, Pirbright in Surrey and a small arms course at Hythe in Kent, he was posted to Borden in Hampshire. (As an aside, my younger son passed his assessment course at Pirbright in 2009 which saw him go on to join the Parachute Regiment, and in the late 1990s I trained at the Hythe ranges whilst a member of a Police firearms unit.)

Jimmy was employed as an instructor at the Artificer Training School at Borden where he held the rank of sergeant. An artificer, which is a job title and not a rank, is given to a member of the armed forces who has the required skills to work with electronic, electrical, electro-mechanical and or mechanical devices. It was in 1954, during the five years he spent there serving with the REME, that he met and married his wife. He was now 25 years of age.

In 1955 Jimmy was on the move again, this time he decided to transfer to the Military Provost Staff Corps and was stationed at Colchester in Essex. He ended up serving with them for seventeen years, during which time he was stationed in Malaya and Hong Kong for three years. On his return to the United Kingdom in 1958 he was posted to the Military Prison at Shepton Mallet in Somerset, where he remained for the following three years.

Planning for the future and looking at life after his time in the Army, Jimmy and his wife decided to purchase a house in Edinburgh, with a view to joining the Scottish Prison Service, but all this changed when two of their children, who were twins and only eighteen months old, died unexpectedly. After talking it over, Jimmy and his wife decided that it would be best that he remain in the Army so that he would eventually have a reasonable pension. In 1972 he reached that milestone when he celebrated twenty-five years' military service.

An interesting discussion took place in the House of Commons about the Military Prison at Shepton Mallet on 6 May 1959, which was during the period Jimmy was serving with the Military Provost Staff Corps. Questions were asked of the then Secretary of State for War, who was also the Member of Parliament for Bedford, Mr Christopher Soames.

A few of the questions and answers would be useful to record as they highlight the standards required to serve with the Military Provost Staff, as well as the number and type of individuals they were tasked with looking after.

The initial question was asked by the MP for Beckenham, Mr Philip Goodhart: '*How many soldiers are now serving sentences of imprisonment or detention in the military detention centre at Shepton Mallet; and how many of these men will be released from the Army at the end of their sentence?*'

Mr Soames replied: '*One hundred and forty-one, all of whom, have or will be discharged from the Army.*'

Mr Charles Simmons, the MP for Brierley Hill, a district in the West Midlands, asked the following question of the Home Secretary: '*What are the staffing levels at Shepton Mallet military prison; what are the qualifications of the staff; and to what extent they are subject to inspection by independent, outside bodies?*'

Mr Soames explained that apart from administrative staff, the Military Provost Staff Corps, provided six officers along with forty-seven warrant officers and non-commissioned officers to look after those who were detained there. *'Members of the Corps are all volunteers from other arms of the Service. They are selected for qualities of authority and leadership; and they have to succeed at an intensive course of training. Inspection is undertaken by military authorities, and there are visits by members of the Prison Commission, whose help and advice we welcome.'*

Mr Goodhart explained that he had recently visited the prison where he met many of the staff, who he said were doing a very difficult job whilst having to working in very depressing surroundings. Mr Simmons posed the question about whether the staff were 'strong-arm men', an inference which could possibly suggest that they were a bit thuggish in the appearance and how they carried out their duties. His comments in part arose from photographs which had appeared in the press, 'some of them were not exactly reassuring.' Mr Simmons eloquently replied.

Mr Soames's reply was immediate and succinct: *'The staff of the prison are certainly not strong-arm men in the sense in which the hon. Member refers, but they are also not weak-arm men.'*

The discussion in its entirety makes for interesting reading. For those wanting to do so, it can be found on Hansard volume 605 pages 368–74.

Jimmy left Shepton Mallet on promotion in 1963 to run the Military Correction Training Centre in Colchester, Essex, where he remained for three years. From there he went out to Singapore where he spent two and a half years, which was also his last foreign posting with the Military Provost Staff Corps. The fact that Jimmy had his wife and three children with him in Singapore, made it an even more enjoyable experience. When they returned from Singapore in 1968 they purchased a house in Colchester for £4,500. The family grew up in Colchester and he retired there in 1972 having served his twenty-five years in the Army. 'On the whole, not a bad life,' Jimmy says.

After a life in the military he applied to join the Police and was employed in a Community Policing role, finally retiring at the age of 60 in 1989. He continued living in Colchester with his wife until she passed away in 2009, which is when Jimmy made the decision to spend his twilight years as a resident of the Royal Hospital Chelsea.

Jimmy has enjoyed his time as an in-pensioner and found life at the hospital an interesting existence. Since his arrival he has been involved at Remembrance Day celebrations at the Royal Albert Hall, Margaret Thatcher's funeral service at St Paul's Cathedral, and he was also part of the Chelsea Pensioners Guard of Honour for her Majesty the Queen's Golden Jubilee celebrations.

In a letter Jimmy had previously sent me, he ended it by saying, 'Not a bad ending in my opinion.' As far as I can see, Jimmy has many years to go before his story finally runs its course.

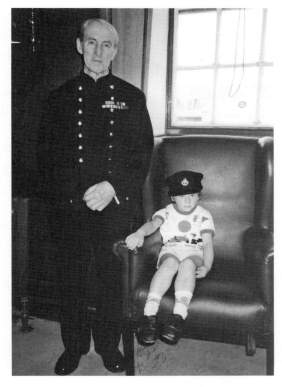

Figure 20: James Parks, in-pensioner (1975–88) and his grandson, Darryl Clarke.

Darryl Clarke is a gardener at the Royal Hospital Chelsea and part of his work is tending to the burial area in the hospital's grounds. Previously, he had worked as a gardener for the Commonwealth War Graves Commission at the Brookwood cemetery in Surrey, which allowed him to tend to the graves of those ex-servicemen and women who are buried there.

Darryl's story is an interesting one because not only has he always wanted to be a gardener, but he also wanted to be a gardener working for the Commonwealth War Graves Commission. He achieved his goal and worked at Brookwood Military Cemetery in Surrey between 2003 and 2004, which allowed him to personally tend the grave of his grandfather, James Parks, who served as a Private (6396368) in the Royal Sussex Regiment.

Working in the grounds of the Royal Hospital Chelsea, also provides him with further fulfilment as he gets to work where his grandfather was an

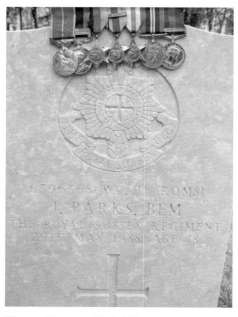

Figure 21: James Parks' Gravestone.

in-pensioner for thirteen years between 1975 and 1988.

James Parks was born in 1910 in Lewes, East Sussex and in 1928, just after his eighteenth birthday, he joined the Army, enlisting in the Royal Sussex Regiment in Chichester. This had a special significance to James, as his own father had served with the same regiment for fourteen years between 1889 and 1903.

During the Second World War he was part of the British Expeditionary Force and was one of the thousands who were evacuated from the beaches of Dunkirk in

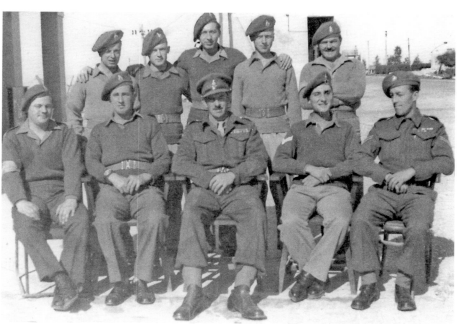

Figure 22: James Parks and some of his colleagues during the Second World War.

May 1940. James's regiment, the Royal Sussex, were part of the 44ᵗʰ Division, and he and his comrades were taken back to England on board HMS *Vivacious*, a V Class Destroyer of the Royal Navy.

HMS *Vivacious* made numerous journeys from the dangerous beaches of Dunkirk to the safety of Dover. On 28 May 1940, she made two trips, evacuating 326 men on the first one and a further 359 on the second. On 30 May she made one journey where she rescued 527 men, once again dropping them off at Dover. On 31 May she was struck by shells fired from German howitzers situated at Bray Dunes, on the coast of northern France, close to the border with Belgium. Fortunately, she hadn't picked up any troops from the beaches, but fifteen of her crew were injured in the bombardment. There was no respite for *Vivacious* for she was back in the thick of things the following day, when she picked up another 427 men from Dunkirk and returned them safely to Dover.

James Parks was safely evacuated from Dunkirk on either 28 or 30 May or 1 June. Later in the war, James and his unit were sent out to North Africa as part of the famous Eighth Army, and from there he was sent to Italy where he found himself embroiled in the fighting at Monte Cassino. It was there, on 16 February 1944, that his war came to an end when he was wounded by shrapnel from a German hand grenade at what was known as Snakeshead Ridge.

On 13 December 1945 he was awarded the British Empire Medal for helping in the wartime evacuation of Greek civilians.

James finished his military career in 1949 at the rank of Warrant Officer Class II, Regimental Quartermaster Sergeant, after twenty-one years' service in the British Army. His desire to become a Chelsea Pensioner arose from having read a book about the Royal Hospital in 1965 and ten years later, he was one of those pensioners whom he had previously read about.

During his thirteen years as an in-pensioner at the hospital, he met many members of the Royal family, including Her Majesty the Queen in 1982.

When James sadly passed away on 25 May 1988, he was given a full military funeral and was buried in the plot set aside for Chelsea Pensioners at the Brookwood Military Cemetery in Surrey.

As for Darryl, he joined the Army Cadet Force, specifically 'C' Company, 3 Troop, of the Army's Royal Logistical Corps in 1998 at Sandown on the

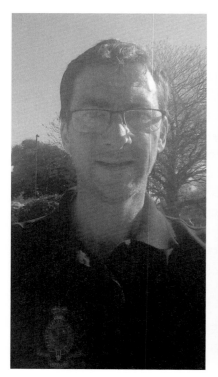 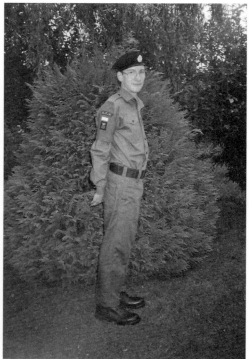

Figure 23: Darryl Clarke.

Isle of Wight. During his training he took part in some twenty-four courses and exercises, which included assault courses and map reading, working alongside regular soldiers from The Princess of Wales's Royal Regiment, which had been born of the amalgamation of the Queen's Regiment and the Hampshire Regiment in 1992. Sadly, his dreams of serving full time in the military were dashed due to an injury which he sustained in July 1998 during training on an Army assault course.

Paul Whittick is an in-pensioner at the Royal Hospital Chelsea and has been since 9 November 2015. His had been a relatively quick process. Having first applied to become a resident of the Royal Hospital in June of that year, he was then invited for a four-day stay, which began on 21 September, and then having liked what he had seen and experienced, just over six weeks later he was in – a fully fledged Chelsea Pensioner.

Paul, who was from humble beginnings as one of eleven children, ten brothers and a sister Margaret, was born in Manchester in 1949. His father had been a military man having served with the King's Own Borderers, so it was a natural assumption that one or more his sons might follow suit. Including Paul, six of his sons went on to enlist in the military, all of them wearing different cap badges.

Paul's choice was the Royal Army Medical Corps which with his previous boyhood experience as a First Aider in the St John Ambulance Brigade, was a natural path to take. When he left school in 1964 at 15 years of age, he enlisted as a boy soldier. Two years later and now 17 years of age, he received his first posting, which was an overseas one, in Aden. This wasn't some nice cushy little posting consisting of sun, sea and sangria, because at the time Paul was stationed in Aden, there was in place an emergency, known as the Aden Emergency, which was also referred to as the Radfan Uprising. It was an insurgency against the territories of South Arabia, which today is known as South Yemen, by members of the National Liberation Front (Yemen) (NLF) and the Front for the Liberation of Occupied South Yemen (FLOSY).

The troubles had started on 14 October 1963 when a suspected member of the pan Arab Nationalist movement, threw a grenade at a group of British officials at Aden Airport. This resulted in a state of emergency being called in the region, which remained in place for the following four years and only came to an end when the British forces withdrew on 30 November 1967.

Paul and his comrades were in as much danger as those serving in infantry regiments, because every time a unit went out on a long-distance patrol they had at least one of the lads from the Royal Army Medical Corps with them. On 9 September 1966 such a patrol was near the town of Mukeiras, about 120 miles from Aden, when one of the vehicles ran over a mine. Corporal 23698404 S.B. Hardwick of the Royal Army Medical Corps was killed in the subsequent explosion.

After Paul had spent time getting acclimatised to his new environment by working at the RAF Hospital in Aden, he went out on his first attachment with a unit of Royal Marines from 45 Commando who were sent on patrol to Dhala, near the Radfan border. Paul recalls the trip as a massive learning curve for the young and relatively inexperienced young soldier he was at the time, and very exciting. *'Exciting times as I recall, night patrols, border patrols and hairy times. It was by far the best learning curve a soldier could have. The Royal Marines of 45 Commando whom I worked with, took me under their wing and I had a baptism of fire from a first-class group of guys. It was an absolute pleasure to have been associated with them. In return I hope that I gave of my best for them.'*

Paul spent the first four years of his Army service stationed in Dhala, near the Radfan border in the Sultanate of Oman. It is also known as the Queen city of the south, and Sharjah, which is one of the Emirates which makes up the United Arab Emirates.

His military service also took him to Germany where he was based at the British Army Camp of Hohne, near Belsen, before being stationed at Münster.

Paul finally left the Army in 1976 because he felt that his career appeared to be stagnating. He took a massive gamble, threw caution to the wind, and decided to buy himself out of the Army, despite not having a clue about what he was going to do next. At the time he wasn't quite sure if he 'was being stupid or brave', but something told him that there was a job out there in civvy street with his name on it, all he had to do was find it.

Back home in England he took himself off to the Job Centre. The person who interviewed him asked what he wanted to do. That was a simple one for Paul to answer, 'anything medical'. 'What about an anatomical pathological technician?' the interviewer asked. 'I can do that,' Paul answered eagerly. After a quick phone call by the Job Centre, Paul had himself an interview to go to within the hour. As he went to leave, the lady who had interviewed him asked what the job entailed; with a wry smile on his face, he replied, 'post-mortems'. As he turned to walk out the door, he saw an uncomfortable grimace appear across her face.

Paul, passed the interview with flying colours and the job was his. He remained there for the next four years, until the desire to do something else, returned. He took another risk, left his job as an anatomical pathological technician and went to college where he studied for a commercial diploma. On completing his studies he spent two years gaining experience as a Fleet Maintenance Administrator.

Whilst in London visiting a friend, he came across one of the numerous free newspapers that can be found discarded on the seats of the tube trains. He flicked through until he came to the jobs section. Amongst the many vacancies, he spotted a post for an Academic Secretary, to a Professor of Immunology, at St Bartholomew's Hospital and the Royal London School of Medicine and Dentistry. *'I just instinctively knew that this was something which I wanted to do, something that I found really appealing and as an added bonus, the pay was far more than I earned as a Fleet Maintenance Administrator.'*

Paul sent a letter and his CV and was invited for an interview where he met Professor Gian Franco Bottazzo and was offered the job. They worked closely together for eight years, during which time Paul was often invited to the professor's London home for social occasions and was even invited to the celebrations for the professor's fiftieth birthday in Venice. Paul's work consisted of typing up drafts of his work for publication in medical magazines, plus acquiring any artwork or images that were required with each submission. He also had to prepare lecture slides for the professor to use at seminars and lectures as he travelled the world talking about his field of expertise.

Sadly, nothing stays the same for ever and one day in 1997, out of the blue, the Professor announced that he was going home to Italy to take up a post working in Rome. Paul was invited to carry on working for him, but unfortunately the 'Italian Job' would only be for three years, which left Paul without the job security he wanted.

Paul's reputation was such that he wasn't short of other job offers once news of Professor Bottazzo's departure became known. One of the opportunities which came his way was an offer from a professor in the Dean's office of the medical facility where Paul was already working. He became the personal assistant to three eminent professors: Professor Nigel Benjamin, a pharmacologist; Professor Peter Koppleman, a consultant in obesity and Professor Irene Leigh, a dermatologist. The job was varied and interesting, especially as it was a time when new teaching practices were being implemented at the Medical School where Paul was working. He remained there for two years before making the decision to leave his job and move back to Cornwall where the pace of life was a lot more sedate.

There was a certain sad irony attached to Paul's decision for wanting to become a Chelsea Pensioner. His father and his six brothers, who served in the Army, would all have liked to have become Chelsea Pensioners, but unfortunately none of them met the criteria. Putting on his scarlet tunic fills Paul with immense pride and every time he does it for his father and brothers, and also for all those who served in the military and never made it back from foreign fields, in both world wars and every other theatre of war, where British soldiers have served. It is a constant reminder to him that somebody's brother, sister, mother or father, served and died, making the ultimate sacrifice in the pursuit of peace.

During his time as an in-pensioner, Paul has had the pleasure of attending many different functions, both in and out of the hospital. Good health permitting, he intends to keep wearing his Scarlets, over the forthcoming years, so that he can inform as many people as possible about the pensioners, what they do, what they stand for and the reasons behind why he chose to wear the famous Scarlet Tunic of the Chelsea Pensioners.

Paul says, *'I came to the Royal Hospital Chelsea for camaraderie, the military ethos, and the hope that I can educate people about this magnificent establishment that has existed for 325 years for the benefit of ex-servicemen who have been broken by war. We that have served will know why we need the Royal Hospital Chelsea, but if you have never served you will never properly understand.'*

As Paul sees it, he just happens to live in the greatest 'Old People's Home', in the world. From the moment he became a Chelsea Pensioner, or as he describes it, 'his final posting' or 'final resting place', he has been cared for both emotionally and physically. The facilities which the hospital provides are second to none. There is an activities and volunteer section which caters for most hobbies from art to pottery, and 'everything in between'. These include, boules, bowls, football, cricket, putting, garden plots, art workshops, hobby rooms for belt making and jewellery workshops, just to mention a few.

The volunteers befriend the pensioners who might just be in need of something as straightforward as company, or somebody to push them round the grounds, or help them with shopping. Paul describes them as being amazing people. As for the hospital's care staff and the sterling job that they do, he highlights that they go far beyond their normal tasks by helping the pensioners in their everyday lives. *'We are without doubt privileged to have such a great group of care staff, from the Matron down, including the housekeepers who do such a great job in keeping this vast place clean. We have a resident doctor and a medical reception team who care for all of our needs.'*

Every day Paul muses about how he gets to eat his meals in the historic Great Hall where they are served by waiters who greet them with a smile and

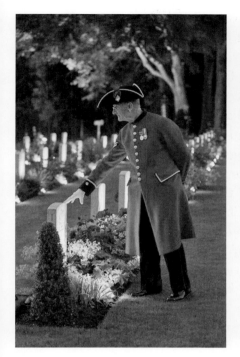
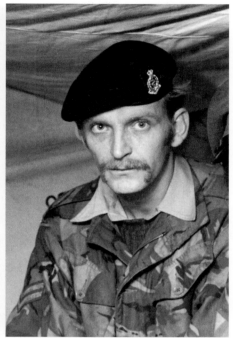

Figure 24: Paul Whittick - Courtesy of Jeremy Selwyn.

Figure 25: Paul Whittick. (Additional Photograph).

a kind word, which usually results in some small talk and a laugh. The porter staff are just the same, always happy to move the pensioners' things around from one place to another, with a smile and some good humoured banter. Every need is catered for from haircuts to podiatrist, by staff that care, and who provide an amazing experience, to those they are charged to look after.

In closing Paul said, *'This is the greatest care home for ex Army personnel of which I am one of the lucky ones to be here. I am proud, privileged and honoured to be a Chelsea Pensioner along with my fellow peers. To all soldiers who made the ultimate sacrifice, Rest in Peace.'*

Marjorie Cole was born in Hull in 1944. Little did she know then the part she was destined to play in the history of the Royal Hospital Chelsea.

We had the pleasure of meeting Marjorie at the Royal Hospital on a bitterly cold winter's morning in January 1918. What made it even more special,

Figure 26: Marjorie Cole. Her two medals, are the General Service Medal, for services in the Malaya Peninsular 1965 - 1966 with a bar for service in Northern Ireland. The other is the Pingat Jasa Medal, awarded by the King and Government of Malaysia (1957 - 1966).

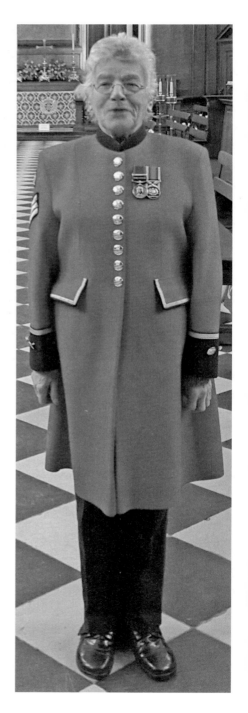

was that it was a chance meeting. We were at the hospital to look through their Second World War diary and to take some pictures for inclusion in this book. As we had arrived early we went about taking the photographs we needed. Our first port of call just happened to be the Wren Chapel, which was built between 1681 and 1687, and that's where we first met the lovely Marjorie. Here is her story in her own words:

'In September 1961, I signed on at the Army Recruiting office in Hull, East Yorkshire to serve for three years in the Women's Royal Army Corps (WRAC). After I had left school at fifteen, and up to enlisting in the WRAC, I'd worked for two years in a large bakery, but it wasn't what I could see me doing for the rest of my days. Life was pretty boring back then, and I had this strong feeling that I needed to get away and explore the world, see new things and meet new people. I didn't want to end up getting married young, like most of my old school friends had.

Having signed on the dotted line and committed myself to the Army for three years, I made my way by train to Lingfield in Surrey in early October 1961, to begin my six-week basic training. That was the start of my military career. I was posted to various places and eventually I ended up as a military chief instructor at the Army School of Catering at Aldershot.

I was very happy with my decision to join the Army, but due to a problem with my back, which required me to undergo two major operations, aged 33 I was medically discharged from the Army in May 1977, after having served for fourteen and a half years. I would have liked to have remained in the

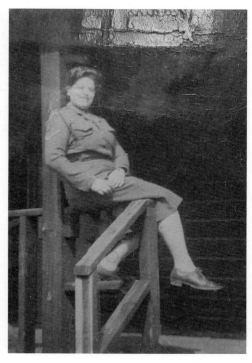

Figure 27: Marjorie Cole at Kingston Gate.

Army, but sadly, it was not to be. But I took with me some good memories of my time serving my Queen and country.

I twice served in Singapore. The first occasion was between 1965 and 1966 and the second was between 1969 and 1971. It is truly a beautiful country. I also served in Northern Ireland between 1972 and 1973.

One funny and slightly embarrassing story I have from my service in the WRAC, took place in November 1971 when I was stationed at Kingston Gate Camp, in Richmond Park, Surrey. It was only a few days away from that year's Remembrance Sunday service, when I looked at the Daily Orders. One of the items included on it was the instruction that "ALL MEDALS WILL BE WORN". Me, being in only my second month of service, decided to approach my Company Sergeant Major to ensure there was no ambiguity about what that order actually meant. "Please Ma'am, does that include my swimming medals?" I can't tell you what her reply was, well I could, but I'm not going to. That's how green I was back then.

When I was discharged from the Army I decided to move back to my native Hull to live with my parents. I continued living with them until in October 1977 when I acquired a flat in the town of Hessle, which is in the East Riding of Yorkshire and five miles west of Kingston-upon-Hull city centre. It sits on the north bank of the Humber Estuary where the Humber Bridge crosses.

I remained living in Hessle – during which time I helped nurse my mother and sister who both subsequently died of cancer – until I became a Chelsea Pensioner in July 2009, only the third woman who was given the honour of becoming one of the hospital's full-time residents, and part of the long history of the Royal Hospital. I have always felt that to be fortunate enough to become a Chelsea Pensioner, to have the opportunity to wear the Queen's uniform again, is a tremendous privilege, as is being an ambassador of the Royal Hospital Chelsea.

Every day here can be a new experience, with the kind of events that a pensioner can take part in or attend. Two of the experiences I have been fortunate enough to be involved in during my time at the hospital have included, taking part in a procession in Westminster Abbey, back in June 2013, to commemorate the 60th anniversary of the Queen's Coronation. It was like living a fairy tale as I remember listening to the original broadcast of the Coronation service on the radio, back in June 1953, when I was only 9 years of age.

The other memorable experience for me, which sticks out from the many which I have had since being at the hospital, was being selected to carry the casket of Margaret Thatcher's ashes from the Vestry into the Chapel of All Saints which is situated in the Margaret Thatcher Infirmary, at her interment service which took place in the hospital's grounds in September 2013.

Since August 2009 I have been a volunteer chapel attendant in the hospital's world famous Wren Chapel, which is a role I enjoy very much indeed, getting as I do, to meet and talk to people from all around the world.'

Chapter 8

Royal Hospital Chelsea Governors

There has been a Board of Commissioners in charge of the hospital since 1702. Its role is to ensure that the hospital is operating as it should be, in relation to the continued care and well-being of the in-pensioners and to look after its many historic buildings. Since 1714 the hospital has also had a governor, or a figurehead, a man in charge.

1686 – 1702: **Colonel Sir Thomas Ogle** became the first Governor of the Royal Hospital on 1 November 1686, a post he held until 16 November 1702. He died just nine days after stepping down from his position.

1702 – 1714: **Colonel John Hales**

1714 – 1720: **Brigadier General Thomas Stanwix** had a distinguished military career, followed by one as a politician, and was the Governor of Gibraltar before he became the Governor of the Royal Hospital Chelsea in 1714.

By the time he was 22 years of age, in 1692, he already held the rank of captain lieutenant in the Hastings Foot Regiment. Although in March of 1702 he became the Member of Parliament for Carlisle, he didn't relinquish his commission in the Army, and the following year in 1703, he took part in the Battle of Caia in Portugal during the War of the Spanish Succession. In 1705 he became the lieutenant governor for his constituency town of Carlisle, which at the time was a major location for the smuggling of goods between England and Scotland. In 1711 he was on the move again, this time to the island of Gibraltar where he became the Governor on 24 January 1711. During his term of office, Spain ceded Gibraltar to Great Britain as part of the Treaty of Utrecht. Thomas Stanwix held the post until 7 August 1713, when he was replaced by General, The Earl of Portmore, David Colyear.

Stanwix's greatest achievement whilst Governor of Gibraltar, appears to have been to make himself richer than he already was. On leaving the island he returned to England and a year later, in 1714, he became the Governor of the Royal Hospital Chelsea, which was an honorary title, he was by then, 44 years of age. This was a position he held for the next six years, but despite this he still found time to become the Mayor of Carlisle for 1715 as well as the Lieutenant of Cumberland, whilst still remaining the MP for Carlisle, until 1721, when he lost his seat. He didn't hang around feeling sorry for himself though, instead in the same year he became the MP for Newport in Wales, but only for a year, before then taking up the same position at Yarmouth in Norfolk. In 1717 he became the Colonel of the Stanwix Regiment of Foot, which would in later years become part of the Suffolk Regiment, whilst in 1721 he also took on the military position of Governor of Kingston-upon-Hull, a role he kept until in his death on 14 March 1725.

1720 – 1722: Lieutenant General Charles Churchill took over as governor of the Royal Hospital Chelsea from Thomas Stanwix in 1720. That he ever reached such lofty heights in British society, is a remarkable achievement taking into account the fact that he was born illegitimately in 1679 to Elizabeth Dodd. Fortunately for Charles and his mother, his father was General Charles Churchill (later to become the Lieutenant of the Tower of London in 1702) which made a massive difference as to how his life turned out. His uncle was John Churchill, 1st Duke of Marlborough.

Charles Churchill served in the British Army during the War of the Spanish Succession, which lasted for more than 12 years, between 1702 and 1714. One of the outcomes of the war was France recognising Britain's sovereignty over the quaintly named, 'Rupert's Land' which was part of British North America.

In 1715 Charles Churchill became the MP for Castle Rising, a parliamentary borough in Norfolk, a position which he held until his death on 14 May 1745. He is reported to have fathered two illegitimate children, a son, with an English actress by the name of Anne Oldfield, and a daughter, Harriet. Once again, being illegitimate didn't do the Churchill family any harm, as in her adult life, Harriet, married Sir Everard Fawkener.

Whilst the Member of Parliament for Castle Rising and the Governor of the Royal Hospital Chelsea, he was still serving in the military and was promoted to the rank of brigadier in 1727 before becoming a Groom of the Bedchamber, which was a position in the Royal Household, on 14 September the same year. It was a role he continued in until 20 January 1746.

1722 – 1740: Lieutenant General William Evans served during the War of Spanish Succession in 1713, as Colonel of Princess Anne of Denmark's Regiment of Dragoons, a position he held until 1735. He was promoted to the rank of lieutenant colonel in 1727, six years later in 1733, he also became the colonel of the Queen's Own Regiment of Horse, a position he held until 1740.

1740 – 1768: Field Marshal Sir Robert Rich, 4th Baronet, was born on 3 July 1685 at Roos Hall, Beccles in Suffolk. He became an ensign in the 1st Regiment of Foot Guards and a lieutenant in the Army in 1700, when he was just 15 years of age.

During the War of the Spanish Succession in Bavaria he fought in the Battle of Schellenberg in July 1704 and at the Battle of Blenheim in August 1704 and was wounded on both occasions.

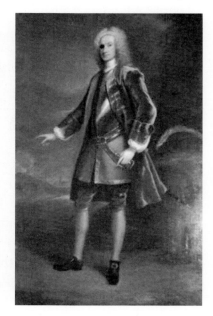

In March 1708 he was promoted to the rank of lieutenant colonel and three months later he was involved in a duel with Sir Edmund Bacon, 4th Baronet. He was wounded, but both men survived.

The last recorded case of two men settling a disagreement between themselves in a pistol duel, was at Priest Hill near Windsor Castle in England, in 1852, ironically involving two Frenchmen. This resulted in the death of French politician, Frederick Cournet, who died the same day of his injuries. The man who fired the fatal shot was fellow French refugee, Emmanuel Barthelemy. He was tried for the capital offence of murder but was acquitted by a jury.

Figure 28: Field Marshal Sir Robert Rich.

In June 1715 Robert Rich was elected as the MP for Dunwich in Suffolk but lost his seat in the General Election of 1722. Two years later he once again became a Member of Parliament, this time for Bere Alston in Devon.

In September 1725 he became the Colonel of Sir Robert Rich's Regiment of Dragoons, and in 1727, and having been the MP for Bere Alston for only four years, he left and became the new MP for the constituency of St Ives, the same year that he was appointed a Groom of the Bedchamber in the Royal household of King George II, a position he held until 1759.

On 15 March 1927 he was promoted to the rank of brigadier general and further promotions followed, including the one that saw him become the colonel of the 4th Regiment Dragoons in May 1733. He reached the rank of lieutenant general on 17 July 1739 and became the Governor of the Royal Hospital Chelsea the following May. An interesting point about Rich is that whilst holding the position of governor, he saw action during the Battle of Dettingen in Bavaria, during the War of the Austrian Succession. He was promoted to the rank of field marshal on 3 December 1757 whilst still the governor of the Royal Hospital Chelsea, a position he held until his death on 1 February 1768.

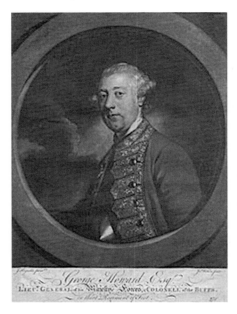

Figure 29: Sir George Howard.

1768 – 1795: **Field Marshal Sir George Howard KB PC** was born on 17 June 1718, the son of Lieutenant General Thomas Howard and his wife Mary.

He served in the British Army for 60 years beginning in 1736, when he was 18 years of age. During his years of military service,he was involved in numerous actions including the Battle of Fontenoy in May 1745 during the War of the Austrian Succession, the Battle of Falkirk Muir on 17 January 1746, the Battle of Culloden on 16 April 1746 during the Jacobite Rising of 1745, the Battle of Lauffield on 2 July 1747 during the War of Austrian Succession and the Battle of Warburg on 31 July 1760 during the Seven Years' War.

On 14 March 1761 he was promoted to the rank of lieutenant general, the same year he became the Member of Parliament for Lostwithiel, in Cornwall. In 1763 his life changed direction once again when he was appointed Knight Commander of the Bath and became the colonel of the 7th (The Queen's Own) Regiment of Dragoons in 1766, he became the Governor of Minorca, a position he held for two years, before he handed over to General John Mostyn in 1768. George Howard returned to England and the same year he became the Governor of the Royal Hospital Chelsea, as well as being elected as the MP for Stamford in Lincolnshire. Neither of these positions resulted in him resigning or retiring from the Army. Quite the opposite in fact, as on 6 September 1777 he was promoted to the rank of General, and in April 1779, he became colonel of the 1st (King's) Dragoon Guards.

What would in today's world be considered way too old to still be serving in any branch of the armed forces, George Howard, was promoted to the rank of field marshal on 18 October 1793, when he was 75 years old. He died on 16 July 1796 at his home in Grosvenor Square, London, whilst still in post as the Governor of the Royal Hospital Chelsea and at the same time also holding the honorary post of Governor of Jersey in 1795.

1795 – 1796: Field Marshal the 1st Marquess Townshend PC was born in London on 28 February 1724, to Charles, 3rd Viscount Townshend and Audrey Ethelreda Townshend. He went on to be educated at Eton College and St John's College, Cambridge.

In 1743 19-year-old George Townshend joined the Army as a volunteer and almost immediately saw action at the Battle of Dettingen in June 1743 during the War of the Austrian Succession. Just two years later in April 1745 he was promoted to the rank of captain in the 7th Regiment of Dragoons and once again saw action whilst fighting in Holland. In April 1946 Townshend fought at the Battle of Culloden which was the final confrontation of the Jacobite rising of 1745. On 2 July 1747, having transferred to the 20th Regiment of Foot some five months earlier as the aide-de-camp to the Duke of Cumberland, he took part in the Battle of Lauffeld during the War of the Austrian Succession.

Whilst still serving in what is now Belgium, he was elected unopposed as the Member of Parliament for Norfolk, even though he wasn't even in the country at the time. As odd as that might appear, it has to be remembered that then only a very small percentage of the population could vote, and all of them were men. Women, regardless of their position in society or how wealthy they might be, were not allowed to vote and only men with money and property rights were eligible to do so.

Townshend was something of a maverick and at times appeared to antagonise his peers and some of those around him. An officer and a gentleman was expected to behave and conduct himself by both the unwritten rules of society and the expectations of their comrades. These were not ideals with which Townshend appeared to concern himself, however, he was a just man who had the well-being of the men under his command at the forefront of his thinking.

On his return to England, he audaciously wrote a pamphlet which was deeply critical of the Duke of Cumberland's military skills, knowledge and abilities. As can be imagined, it was not a piece of literature that was well received by the duke or his extremely influential friends and family, his father being King George II. He was the youngest of the king's three sons.

There may have been some substance to Townshend's opinion of his superior officer, as the Duke of Cumberland's military career, wasn't particularly outstanding apart from his victory at the Battle of Culloden and his brutal putting down of the Jacobite Rising.

Townshend argued in parliament that a court martial should be responsible for Army discipline and not a man's commanding officer, whose decision-making process might inevitably be affected by wishing to set an example to the other troops under his command, which might not have a favourable outcome for the man concerned.

George Townshend was promoted to the rank of colonel on 6 May 1758. In September 1759 he found himself in Canada, having to take command of British forces at the Battle of the Plains of Abraham, after his commanding officer, General James Wolfe, was killed in action on 13 September 1759, having been shot three times whilst leading his men in an attack against the French. General Wolfe's second-in-command Robert Monkton was wounded and also put out of the fight, leaving Townshend to take the lead. He once again blotted his copybook by drawing a caricature of the much loved and admired General Wolfe, a man who for some reason Townshend held in contempt.

He then fought at the Battle of Villinghausen which took place over 15 and 16 July 1761, during the Seven Years' War, by which time he had been promoted to the rank of major general, and was in command of 28th Regiment of Foot. His promotions continued. On 2 February 1773, whilst a lieutenant general, he fought a duel with the 1st Earl of Bellomont, Charles Coote. Townshend was uninjured having shot Coote in the groin.

At 71 years of age he became Governor of the Royal Hospital Chelsea and on 30 July the following year, by then, 72 years of age, he was promoted to the rank of field marshal, not long before he retired from the Army. It would appear that he retired from the Army at around the time he stood down as the hospital's governor.

He died on 14 September 1807, aged 83, at his home at Raynham Hall, Norfolk.

1796 – 1804: General Sir William Fawcett KCB was born in 1727. Unlike many of his contemporaries, he was not from a university background, having received his education at Bury Grammar School in Lancashire. His military career began in 1748 when he was commissioned into the 33rd Foot. He went on to serve in Germany as the aide-de-camp to the Marquess of Granby, during the Seven Years' War as well as the American Revolutionary War, which took place between 19 April 1775 and 3 September 1783.

It was in his retirement from the Army that he took up the position of the Governor of the Royal Hospital Chelsea in 1796. It appears to have been common practice then to have held many positions at the same time, as can be seen by the list below.

Governor of Gravesend and Tilbury 1776 – 1796

Colonel of the 15th (Yorkshire East Riding) Regiment of Foot 1778 – 1792

Adjutant General 1781 – 1799

Colonel of the 3rd (Prince of Wales's) Dragoon Guards 1792 – 1804

Governor, Royal Hospital Chelsea 1796 – 1804

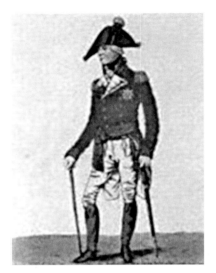

Figure 30: Sir David Dundas.

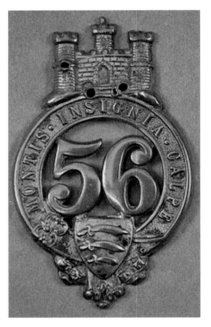

Figure 31: Badge of 56th Foot.

1804 – 1820: **General Sir David Dundas GCB** was born in Edinburgh in 1735 and grew up a proud Scotsman. His father, Robert Dundas, was a well-off merchant, affluent enough to be able to enrol his son at the prestigious Royal Military Academy at Woolwich. On 1 March 1755, at 20 years of age, he graduated from the Academy as a lieutenant fire worker in the Royal Artillery. This rank came next in line after that of a lieutenant and second lieutenant, but was abolished altogether by the Royal Artillery in 1771.

Less than a year after his graduation from the Academy, he transferred to the 56th (West Essex) Regiment of Foot with a promotion to the rank of lieutenant and served with them during the Seven Years' War. Their headquarters garrison was located at Warley Barracks, just outside Brentwood, Essex.

He saw action at the French ports of St Malmo and Cherbourg and in numerous other battles including, on 11 September 1758, the Battle of Saint Cast in France.

On 21 March 1759 he was promoted to the rank of captain and transferred to the 15th Dragoons, with whom he fought at the Battle of Warburg in present day Germany on 31 July 1760; the Battle of Kloster Kampen on 15 October 1760 and the Battle of Villinghausen, which took place over 15 and 16 July 1761. All three battles were part of the Seven Years' War, which in its simplest terms, was Great Britain and her Allies against France and her Allies, but was a global conflict, quite possibly the first ever World War. Dundas was also present at the capture of Havana, Cuba in August 1762.

He was promoted to the rank of brevet colonel on 12 February 1782, but eighteen months later he took up a position as an instructor involved in officer training. So dedicated was he to his new role that he took to writing tactical manuals, the first of which was entitled *Principles of Military Movements* which was published in 1788. Some of the content would have no doubt been based on his own experiences in battle, but also from what he encountered whilst observing Prussian military manoeuvres in Silesia in 1784.

Dundas, having been promoted to the rank of general in 1802, was made Governor of the Royal Hospital Chelsea on 3 April 1804, a position he held until his death on 18 February 1820. He died at the hospital and is buried in the grounds.

Having led men into battle, watched them die, and suffer from the infliction of hideous wounds, he was certainly of the right calibre to hold the position of Governor of the Royal Hospital Chelsea. He was a man who fully understood the plight of the men that he now found himself in charge of, a true leader.

1820 – 1837: **Field Marshal Sir Samuel Hulse GCH,** was born on 27 March 1746, the second son of Sir Edward Hulse, 2nd Baronet, and his wife, Hannah. On 17 December 1761 he was commissioned as an ensign in the 1st Regiment of Foot Guards. The rank of 'ensign' indicated a junior rank and was in later years replaced by the rank of second lieutenant.

He was deployed for his first active duty, not on some foreign battlefield to fight for the honour of his king and country, but on the streets of London at the time of the Gordon Riots which took place in May and June of 1780. The protest was over official discrimination against Roman Catholics in Great Britain. But those marching on Parliament were in the main Protestants who were complaining about the introduction of the Papists Act 1778, whose purpose it was to mitigate some of these restrictions. The president of the Protestant Association of London, was Lord George Gordon, hence the phrase, 'the Gordon Riots'.

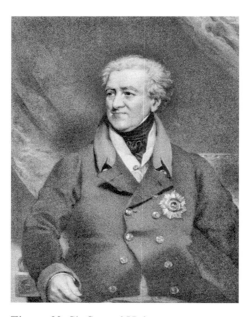

Figure 32: Sir Samuel Hulse.

The first march took place on 29 May 1780 and its target was the House of Commons; there they delivered a petition, demanding that the Act be repealed. On 2 June 1780 a crowd, estimated to be in the region of some 50,000, marched on the Houses of Parliament.

The riots continued over the next few days, becoming worse as time went on. The situation became so bad that troops were called in to deal with the situation and an order was issued that forbade people to mingle in groups of four or more and not disperse when instructed to do so. Troops opened fire killing 285 people and wounding a further 200, whilst a further 450 rioters were arrested. Of these, between twenty and thirty who were tried and found guilty, were executed. It was not a good day in British history and, as news of the riot and its final outcome became widely known, one that damaged the nation's reputation on the world stage.

Ironically the Lord Mayor of London, Mr Brackley Kennett, was convicted of criminal negligence and fined £1,000, for not reading the Riot Act out aloud.

The riots came at the time of the American War of Independence, which led some elements of British society to believe that the two were somehow connected, which they were not, and that the riots were a foreign attempt to destabilise Britain, making her vulnerable to an invasion by a European neighbour.

Samuel Hulse also saw active service during the Flanders Campaign during the French Revolutionary Wars, as well as the Anglo-Russian invasion of Holland. He was appointed as the Lieutenant Governor of the Royal Hospital Chelsea in 1806, whilst continuing to rise through the military ranks. He was knighted in 1821.

Remarkably, by today's standards at least, he received his last promotion on the coronation of King William IV on 22 July 1830, when at 84 years of age, he became a field marshal. He died at the Royal Hospital Chelsea on 1 January 1837.

1837 – 1849: **General Sir Edward Paget GCB** was born on 3 November 1775, the fourth son of Henry Paget, 1st Earl of Uxbridge. His military career began as a cornet, which was the lowest grade a commissioned officer could be at the time, in the 1st Regiment of

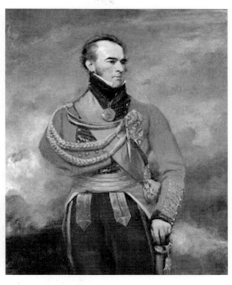

Figure 33: Sir Edward Paget.

Life Guards in 1792 when he was 17 years of age. Four years later he was elected as the Member of Parliament for Caernarvon Boroughs in Wales, making him one of the youngest ever MPs. He held the seat for the following ten years.

He served in the Peninsular War that took place between 1807 and 1814, which was part of the Napoleonic Wars. It refers to the Iberian Peninsula, which was fought over by the Allied powers of Britain, Spain, and Portugal and Napoleon's Empire.

Edward Paget's part in all of this was that he commanded the reserve at the Battle of Corunna in 1809 and conducted the advance to the Portuguese city of Oporto later the same year. He had the distinction of having been captured by French cavalry in 1812 and held as a prisoner until the war ended two years later.

Between 1816 and 1821 he was part of the Royal Household as Groom of the Bedchamber to King George IV. The years between 1822 and 1825 saw him serve in different capacities ranging from, Governor of Ceylon, Commander-in-Chief, India, as well as conducting the Burmese Campaigns of 1824/1825.

He became the Governor of the Royal Military College at Sandhurst in 1826 and from 1837 until 1842 he was the Governor of the Royal Hospital Chelsea. He died on 13 May 1849.

1842 – 1846: General Sir William H. Clinton KCB KCH who was born on 23 December 1769, was the elder son of General Sir Henry Clinton. He was educated at Eton before joining the 7th Light Dragoons and was quickly promoted. A close associate of the Duke of York, he served him as aide-de-camp and military secretary, undertaking several foreign missions, including Governor of Madeira and Lieutenant General of Ordnance. He was MP for East Retford, Nottinghamshire until 1796 and again in 1806, first for the Boroughbridge constituency and later for Newark, until he retired from the Commons in 1829. He died on 15 February 1846. He was Governor of the Royal Hospital Chelsea from 1842 until his death.

1849 – 1849: General Sir George Anson GCB, was only Governor of the Royal Hospital Chelsea for a period of six months, between May and his death at the hospital on 4 November 1849, the shortest reign of any of the hospital's governors.

Having become a soldier at just 17 years of age in 1786, he went on to serve in the British Army in both the French Revolutionary Wars of 1792 to 1802, and the Peninsular War, from 1808 to 1814, where he gained the reputation of being a fine officer.

Outside of his military achievements he was also the MP for Lichfield in Staffordshire between 1806 to 1841, and another who had served as part of the Royal Household as Groom of the Bedchamber to Prince Albert, for five years between 1836 and 1841.

1849 – 1856: General Sir Colin Halkett GCB GCH. His military service included the Peninsular War (1808–1814) and the Hundred Days from Napoleon's escape from Elba to the Battle of Waterloo on 18 June 1815, during which he was wounded four times.

He became Lieutenant Governor of Jersey from 1821 and was appointed Governor of the Royal Hospital Chelsea in 1849, a position he held until his death in 1856.

1856 – 1868: **Field Marshal Sir Edward Blakeney GCB GCH PC** was born on 26 March 1778 in Newcastle-upon-Tyne, the fourth son of Colonel William Blakeney and his wife Sarah. He began his military service on 28 February 1794 when he was commissioned as a cornet in the 8th Light Dragoons. His final promotion to that of field marshal, took place on 9 November 1862, when he was 84 years of age.

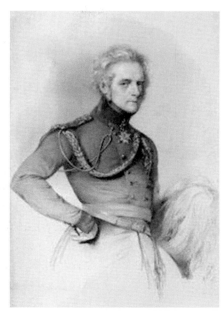

During his military service he had taken part in the French Revolutionary Wars, the Peninsular War, as well as the War of 1812 between Britain and America and their respective allies.

Figure 34: Sir Edward Blakeney.

He became the Governor of the Royal Hospital Chelsea on 25 September 1856 and died there on 2 August 1868, aged 90.

1868 – 1870: **Field Marshal Sir Alexander Woodford KCB KCMG** was born in Welbeck Street, London on 15 June 1782. His parents were Lieutenant Colonel John Woodford and Lady Susan Gordon. He was educated at Winchester College and the Royal Military College at Woolwich.

His military service began when he was commissioned as an ensign, a junior officer, into the 9th (East Norfolk) Regiment of Foot. He went on to serve during the French Revolutionary Wars, the Napoleonic Wars, and also took part in the Battle of Waterloo.

His military service spanned both the decades and centuries, between 1794 and 1843, when he retired from active military service. Despite this he was still promoted to the rank of general on 20 June 1854, and further promoted to the rank of field marshal, on 1 January 1868, twenty-three years after he had retired from active service. He became Governor of the Royal Hospital Chelsea in August 1868. He died on 26 August 1870, in the

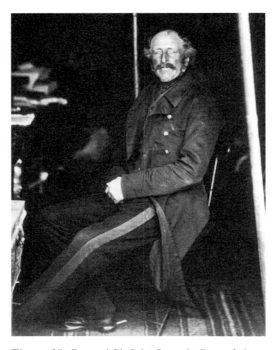

Figure 35: General Sir John Lysaght Pennefather.

Governor's residence at the hospital and was buried at the nearby Kensal Green Cemetery.

1870 – 1872: **General Sir John Lysaght Pennefather GCB**, was born on 9 September 1798, the third son of the Reverend John Pennefather and his wife Elizabeth, the family being well established in Ireland.

His military career began on 14 January 1818, when he became a cornet in the 7th Dragoon Guards, but it would be another twenty-five years before he would experience active service for the first time at the Battle of Miani (or Meeanee), which took place on 17 February 1843, in what is now Pakistan, but was then known as Sindh. History has recorded it as a remarkable achievement, as the British forces numbered just 2,800 men of the British East India Company, whilst their Indian enemy numbered some 30,000 men.

Another notable action he fought in was the Battle of Inkerman during the Crimean War on 5 November 1854. It is said that on a grey and foggy day, Pennefather, who was in command of a division of some 3,000 men, outwitted and defeated a much larger Russian Army, of 35,000 in number.

He was Colonel of the 22nd (The Cheshire) Regiment of Foot between 1860 and 1872, and became the Governor of the Royal Hospital Chelsea in 1870, a position he held until his death on 9 May 1872. He was buried at the Brompton cemetery.

1872 – 1874: **Lieutenant General Sir Sydney Cotton GCB** was born on 2 December 1792, the second son of Henry Calveley Cotton and his wife Matilda.

He joined the British Army in 1810 as a cornet in the 22nd Light Dragoons. He served in India twice, firstly between 1810 and 1835. He then went to Australia, where he served for the following seven years, before returning to India for a second time, where he stayed until 1863. This included the period of the Indian Mutiny between 1857 and 1858.

He became Governor of the Royal Hospital Chelsea in 1872, a position he held until his death, aged 81, on 19 February 1874.

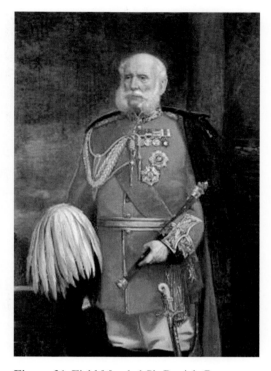

Figure 36: Field Marshal Sir Patrick Grant.

1874 – 1895: **Field Marshal Sir Patrick Grant GCB GCMG** was born on 11 September 1804 in Auchterblair, Scotland, the second son of Major John Grant and his wife Anna Trapaud.

He began his military career at the tender age of 16, when he became an ensign in the Bengal Native Infantry on 16 July 1820, but it would be another twenty-three years before he saw any real action. Here is a list of all of the battles that Grant was involved in:

Battle of Maharajpore – 29 December 1943, Battle of Mudki – 18 December 1845, Battle of Ferozeshah – 21/22 December 1845, Battle of Sobraon – 10 February 1846, Battle of Chillianwala – 13 January 1849, Battle of Gujrat – 21 February 1849.

He was appointed Governor of Malta in 1867 and was promoted to the rank of general on 19 November 1870. Having served in the Indian Army for 57 years, he was placed on the retired list on 1 October 1877, yet still promoted to field marshal six years later on 24 June 1877.

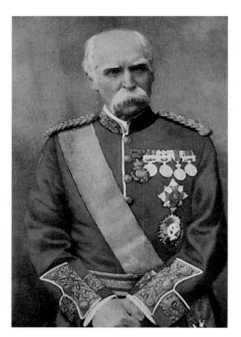

Figure 37: Field Marshal Sir Donald Martin Stewart.

He became the Governor of the Royal Hospital Chelsea in February 1874, a position which continued until his death there on 24 June 1895 when he was 90 years of age. He was buried at Brompton Cemetery.

1895 – 1900: **Field Marshal Sir Donald Martin Stewart, 1st Baronet, GCB GCSI CIE** was born in Moray in Scotland on 1 March 1824, the son of Ronald and Flora Stewart. He went on to study at Aberdeen University.

His military service began at just 16 years of age, when he was commissioned as an ensign in the 9th Bengal Native Infantry on 12 October 1840. He went on to have a remarkable career, taking part in both the Indian Rebellion of 1857 as well as the Second Anglo–Afghan War, 1878 – 1880. During the latter 1,850 British soldiers were killed in action or subsequently died of their wounds, while 8,000 men died of disease.

Other notable positions that he held included being made the Commandant of the Andaman Islands Penal Colony at Port Blair in 1872 and he was present when one of the inmates, Sher Ali Afridi, assassinated the British Viceroy of India, Lord Mayo, by stabbing him with a knife on 8 February 1872. The subsequent inquiry exonerated Stewart from any blame in Lord Mayo's death.

In October 1880 he became a military member of the Council of the Governor General of India, and in April 1881 he was promoted to Commander-in-Chief India.

He became Governor of the Royal Hospital Chelsea in 1895, a position that he held until his death in Algeria on 26 March 1900.

1901 – 1904: **Field Marshal Sir Henry Wylie Norman GCB GCMG GIE** was born in London on 2 December 1826, the son of a merchant, James Norman and his wife, Charlotte.

Having been commissioned as an ensign in the 1st Bengal Native Infantry on 1 March 1844, he went on to serve in the Indian Army for the next 60 years. In doing so he was involved in the Second Anglo–Sikh War of 1848/1849, the Santhal Rebellion of 1855 and the Indian Mutiny of 1857/58.

In January 1862 he became the Military Secretary to the Indian Government and by September 1863 he had returned to England and was made aide-de-camp to Queen Victoria. In 1883 he became

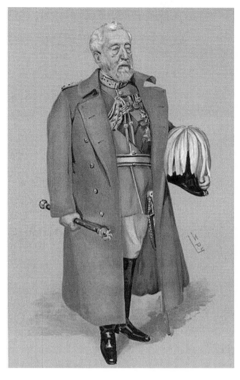

Figure 38: Sir Henry Wylie Norman.

the Governor of Jamaica and in 1889 the Governor of Queensland in Australia, although when he was offered the opportunity to become Viceroy of India in 1893, he declined.

In April 1901 he accepted the position of Governor of the Royal Hospital Chelsea, a position he retained until his death at the hospital on 26 October 1904. During his time as governor at Chelsea, he was promoted to field marshal on 26 June 1902.

1905 – 1912: **Field Marshal Sir George White VC GCB OM GCSI GCMG GCIE GCVO** was born on 6 July 1835 in Ireland. His father, James Robert White, was the Surgeon-General to the British Forces in Ireland. George passed out from the Royal Military College, Sandhurst, on 4 November 1853, and was commissioned as an ensign in the 27th (Inniskilling) Regiment of Foot.

During the course of his fifty-four years of military service with the British Army, George White served in the Indian Mutiny, the Second Anglo-Afghan War, the Third Anglo-Burmese War, the Madhist War and the Second Boer War.

In May 1900 he was appointed as the Governor of Gibraltar, before becoming the Governor of the Royal Hospital Chelsea on 17 June 1905. He died there on 24 June 1912.

He is the only Governor of the Hospital to have been awarded the Victoria Cross. The citation for his acts of bravery reads as follows.

For conspicuous bravery during the engagement at Charasiah on 6 October 1879, when, finding that the artillery and rifle fire failed to dislodge the enemy from a fortified hill which it was necessary to capture. Major White led an attack upon it in person. Advancing with two companies of his regiment, and climbing from one steep ledge to another, he came across a body of the enemy, strongly posted, and outnumbering his force by about 8 to 1. His men being much exhausted, and immediate action being necessary, Major White took a rifle, and going on by himself, shot the leader of the enemy. This act so intimidated the rest that they fled round the side of the hill, and the position was won.

Again, on 1 September 1880 at the Battle of Candahar, Major White, in leading the final charge, under a heavy fire from the enemy, who held a strong position and were supported by two guns, rode straight up to within a few yards of them, and seeing the guns, dashed forward and secured one, immediately after which the enemy retired.

White's Victoria Cross is on display at the Gordon Highlanders Museum, Aberdeen in Scotland.

1912 – 1931: General Sir Neville Lyttelton GCB GCVO PC was born in Hagley, Worcestershire on 28 October 1845, the son of the 4th Baron Lyttelton and his wife Mary. After having been educated at Eton College, Neville Lyttelton was commissioned into the Rifle Brigade.

As a young and inexperienced officer, he was sent to Canada where his input was more in a secretarial sense, than a hands-on military one, although

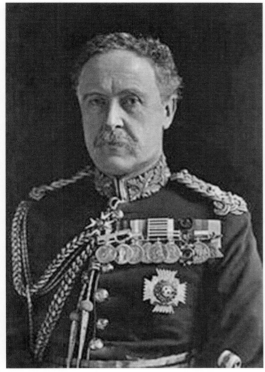

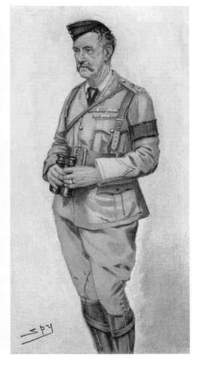

Figure 39a: Neville Lyttelton.
(Caricature).

Figure 39: Neville Lyttelton.

this didn't stop him from rising through the ranks. In 1880 he became the private secretary to the Secretary of State for War, Hugh Childers, who went on to produce what became known as the Childers Reforms of 1881.

He took part in defeating the Fenian Raids in Canada 1866. He acted as aide-de-camp to General Sir John Adye during the Anglo-Egyptian War in 1882, and he saw action during the Battle of Tel-el-Kebir on 13 September 1882, for which his actions were mentioned in despatches. He led the 2nd Brigade at the Battle of Omdurman, during the Mahdist War, in September 1898.

By the time of the Second Boer War in South Africa, between 1899 and 1902, he was in command of the 4th Division when they were engaged at the Battle of Spion Kop in January 1900, the Battle of Vaal Krantz in February 1900 and the Relief of Ladysmith later that month. He went on to hold numerous commands during the course of his 47 years of distinguished service in the British Army, including Commander-in-Chief, Ireland and Chief of the General Staff.

He continued his military service in different guises until his retirement on 10 August 1912, becoming Governor of the Royal Hospital that day at the insistence of King George V. He died whilst still in post, at the hospital on 6 July 1931.

1931 – 1938: **General Sir Walter Pipon Braithwaite GCB** was born in Alne, North Yorkshire on 11 November 1865. The youngest of twelve children, his father was the Reverend William Braithwaite and his mother was Laura Elizabeth Pipon. He studied at the Royal Military Academy, Sandhurst and was commissioned as a lieutenant in the Somerset Light Infantry in 1886. He first saw action during the Second Boer War of 1899–1902, at the battles of Ladysmith, Spion Kop, Vaal Krantz and Tugela Heights, being mentioned in despatches on three occasions.

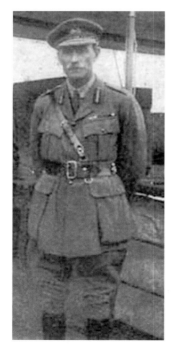

During the First World War he took part in the ill-fated Gallipoli campaign as Chief of Staff, arriving there on 13 March 1915. Regarded as 'arrogant and incompetent' by the Australian troops, he was subsequently dismissed from this position, but on the Western Front he was credited as a competent commander.

The following year saw him having to deal with his own personal grief when his son, Lieutenant Valentine Ashworth Braithwaite MC of the 1st Battalion, Somerset Light Infantry, was killed in action on 2 July 1916, the second day of the Battle of the Somme. He was just 20 years of age. and Sir Walter was understandably devastated by his only son's death.

In January 1917 he was sent to France as part of the 62nd Division where he was involved in the Battle of Arras and the German offensive actions at Bullecourt and Cambrai. He later

Figure 40: General Sir Walter Braithwaite.

went on to command both the IX and XII Army Corps as well as the 9th Army Tank Corps, during the latter stages of the war.

After the signing of the Armistice on 11 November 1918 he remained in the Army at the rank of lieutenant colonel, undertaking many different roles, including in 1928, arranging the funeral of Field Marshal Douglas Haig. He retired from the Army in 1931, the same year in which he was appointed as the Governor of the Royal Chelsea Hospital, a position he held until 1938.

If ever a man was qualified to hold such a position it was Sir Walter Braithwaite, having seen at first hand the death and carnage that went hand in hand with being a front-line soldier. It is quite possible that some of the Chelsea Pensioners who were in-pensioners during his period of tenure, had fought with him during the Boer War.

He died at his home in Rotherwick, Hampshire on 7 September 1945 at the age of 79.

1938 – 1943: General Sir Harry Knox KCB DSO was born on 5 November 1873. He was commissioned into the Northamptonshire Regiment on 26 August 1895 and his first experience of active service came between 1897 and 1898 when he was serving on the North-West Frontier, the border between Afghanistan and what is today, Pakistan, where he was involved in numerous different military operations.

During the First World War he was part of the British Expeditionary Force, and was awarded the Distinguished Service Order in 1917. He was also awarded the *Chevalier Ordre National de la Légion d'Honneur*, as well as the *Croix de Guerre* with Gold Star.

After the war he remained in the military in different capacities. He was aide-de-camp to His Majesty King George V between 1925 and 1926. He held the office of Lieutenant of the Tower of London between 1933 and, 1935, the same year in which he received his knighthood.

1943 – 1949: General Sir Clive Liddell KCB CMG CBE DSO was born in Huddersfield, Yorkshire. He enrolled at the Royal Military College, Sandhurst and joined the Army in 1902. During the First World War he served as Assistant Adjutant and Quartermaster General at the War Office. He remained in the military after the end of the First World War and in 1927 he attended the newly formed Imperial Defence College, at 9 Buckingham Gate, London. Winston Churchill had been in part responsible for recommending the formation of such a college back in 1922.

For the first two years of the Second World War he was the Governor of Gibraltar. On his return to England he served as the Inspector General for Training between 1941 and 1942, before retiring in 1943, the same year he became the Governor of the Royal Hospital Chelsea.

1949 – 1956: **General Sir Bernard Paget GCB MC** was born in Oxford on 15 September 1887. He attended the Royal Military College, Sandhurst, between 1905 and 1907 and, having successfully passed his course, he was commissioned as a second lieutenant into the Oxfordshire and Buckinghamshire Light Infantry in November 1907.

He first went out to the Western Front in May 1915 where he was adjutant to his regiment's newly formed 5th (Service) Battalion. By all accounts he was a brave individual, being mentioned in despatches

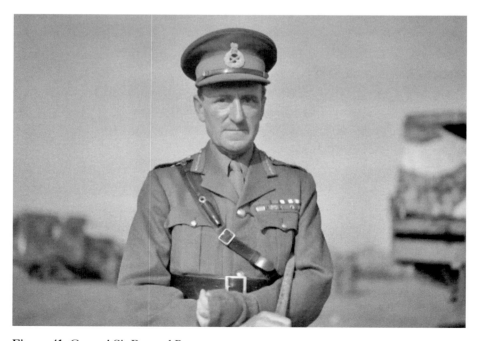

Figure 41: General Sir Bernard Paget.

on four occasions and wounded five times. He was also awarded the Military Cross in November 1915 and the Distinguished Service Order in January 1918.

In the post war years he remained in the Army and at the beginning of the Second World War he was the Commandant of the Staff College at Camberley. During the Second World many of his postings were within the United Kingdom, although in January 1944 he became Commander-in-Chief, Middle East Command, a position he held until October 1946 on his retirement from the Army.

His younger son, Lieutenant Tony Paget, who served with the 1st Battalion, Oxford and Buckinghamshire Light Infantry, the same regiment as his father, died of his wounds on 5 March 1945, during the Battle of the Reichswald, also known as Operation Veritable. He was posthumously awarded the Distinguished Service Order for his actions during the battle.

General Paget died on 16 February 1961.

1956 – 1961: General Sir Cameron Nicholson GCB KBE DSO (Bar) MC (Bar), was born on 30 June 1898. He was commissioned into the Royal Artillery in 1915 and served during the First World War, being awarded the Military Cross twice for his actions in 1918.

During the post war years he became an instructor at the Royal Military Academy, Woolwich, between 1927 and 1930. From 1931 to 1932, he attended the Staff College at Camberley, and between 1938 and 1939, he returned to the Staff College as an instructor.

He served during the Second World War and was awarded the Distinguished Service Order, twice in 1940. As the war continued he proved to be an effective leader both in North Africa against the Germans and in Burma against the Japanese. There is a photograph which is part of the Imperial War Museum's collection which shows a Japanese officer, Captain Tomeichi Okazaki, surrendering his sword to the then Major General Cameron Nicholson in September 1945 at an official ceremony at Johore Bahru, Malaya.

Other awards included being mentioned in despatches, the Silver Star, awarded for valour in combat, and Officer of the Legion of Merit, which is awarded for exceptional meritorious conduct in the performance of outstanding services and achievements; both awards are United States decorations.

He was aide-de-camp to Queen Elizabeth II from 1954 to 1956, retiring from the Army at that time. He died on 7 July 1979 aged 81.

1961 – 1969: **General Sir Frank Simpson GCE KCB DSO** was born on 21 March 1899. He attended the Royal Military Academy at Woolwich, after which he was commissioned into the Royal Engineers in 1916, when he was just 17 years of age. He served throughout the First World War, both in France and Belgium.

On the outbreak of the Second World War he was sent to France and Belgium with the British Expeditionary Force. He took part in the Battle of Arras on 21 May 1940, which was a failed British and French counter-attack to try and break through the German lines. Shortly after this he found himself on the beaches of Dunkirk and was one of those safely evacuated back to the UK. Soon after he arrived home, he became the Chief of Staff to General Montgomery, before moving on to the War Office in 1942. He remained in the Army after the war, eventually retiring in 1954, having served in the British Army for 38 years. He died in 1986 aged 87.

1969 – 1975: **General Sir Charles Phibbs Jones GCB CBE MC** was born in 1906 and served in the British Army between 1925 and 1967. The start of his military career began with his commission into the Royal Engineers.

His service in the Second World War initially saw him sent out to France and Belgium with the British Expeditionary Force in 1940. After being evacuated from the beaches of Dunkirk and making it safely back to the UK, he became an instructor at the Staff College, followed by becoming a General Staff Officer. In 1945 he was sent to Malaya where he became Chief of Staff Malaya Command. In September 1945 he accepted the official surrender of General Kitsuju Ayabe, who had been the Deputy Chief of Staff for the Southern Expeditionary Army Group, stationed in Singapore up until February 1944, when he was badly injured in an airplane crash, and spent the rest of the war assigned to staff duty in Tokyo.

After the war Charles Jones remained in the Army and undertook many different roles, operationally, training and instructing others, with the benefit of his own experiences to assist him in each case. He retired in 1967 after having served in the Army for 42 years. He died on 4 January 1988 aged 81.

1975 – 1981: General Sir Anthony Read GCB CBE DSO MC was born in London on 10 September 1913. He attended the Royal Military College, Sandhurst, and was then commissioned into the Oxfordshire and Buckinghamshire Regiment in 1934. He served during the Second World War when he was awarded the Military Cross whilst fighting against the Italians in East Africa in 1941. He was further awarded the Distinguished Service Order for his service in Burma in March 1945, when in charge of the 1st Gambia Regiment.

After the war Read remained in the Army carrying out a variety of roles, working in Cyprus, as the Commandant of the School of Infantry in Warminster, the Commandant of the Royal College of Defence Studies and aide–de–camp to the Queen from 1971 to 1973. He retired from the British Army in 1974 and died on 22 September 2000.

1981 – 1987: General Sir Robert Cyril Ford GCB CBE was born in Devon on 29 December 1923. He was commissioned into the Royal Armoured Corps in 1943 and before the war was over he had served in North West Europe.

He remained in the Army after the war until retiring in 1981. On 29 July 1971 he became the Commander Land Forces for Northern Ireland, the Bloody Sunday shootings took place during his tenure. In 1973 he became the commandant in charge of the Royal Military Academy at Sandhurst, and he finished his military service by being the aide–de–camp to the Queen between 1980 and 1981. He died on 24 November 2015 aged 91.

1987 – 1993: General Sir Roland Guy GCB CBE DSO was born on 25 June 1928 in Sringar, Kashmir. He studied at the Royal Military Academy at Sandhurst and on the successful completion of his course in 1948, he was commissioned into the King's Royal Rifle Corps. He served in Kenya during the Mau Mau Rising that lasted for eight years between

1952 and 1960, the Indonesia–Malaysia Confrontation between 1963 and 1966, and the Northern Ireland Troubles in 1972, for which he was awarded the Distinguished Service Order. He was another of the long list of men who had been appointed aide-de-camp to the Queen (1984), en route to becoming the Governor of the Royal Hospital Chelsea. He died on 13 December 2005.

1993 – 1999: General Sir Brian Leslie Graham Kenny GCB CBE was born on 18 June 1934. He went on to serve in the British Army for 39 years from 1954 until 1993. His military service had seen him working at the Ministry of Defence in 1984 as the Director of Army Staff Duties. In 1987 he became General Officer Commanding British Forces on the Rhine in Germany, and the Deputy Supreme Allied Commander Europe in 1990 – a substantial and impressive CV. He died on 19 June 2017, aged 83.

1999 – 2006: General Sir Jeremy Mackenzie GCB OBE DL was born in Nairobi, Kenya on 11 February 1941 and began his military career, aged 18, in 1959. On the successful completion of his course, he was commissioned into the 1st Battalion, Queen's Own Highlanders and sent to Singapore. He took part in putting down the Brunei Rebellion in 1962. He served in Northern Ireland during the Troubles and was present at the Warren Point Massacre in Northern Ireland on 27 August 1979, which resulted in the deaths of eighteen young British soldiers, with a further six who were wounded.

The IRA's South Armagh Brigade ambushed the British soldiers with two large roadside bombs. The first blew up part of a British Army convoy, whilst the second bomb was aimed at reinforcements who were sent to the scene to deal with the aftermath of the initial explosion. The attack happened on the same day that the IRA assassinated Lord Louis Mountbatten.

Jeremy Mackenzie, who was second-in-command of the Queen's Own Highlanders at the time of the Warren Point Massacre, had to take command of the Highlanders, when their commanding officer was killed in the ambush.

In 1994 he was promoted to the rank of general and given the post of Deputy Supreme Allied Commander Europe, with responsibility for the co-ordination of the 52,000 troops from the thirty-four nations who had sent peace-keeping troops to Bosnia and Herzegovina.

He was appointed aide-de-camp to Queen Elizabeth between 1992 and 1996. He retired from the Army in 1999 after having served in the British Army for 40 years.

2006 – 2011: Field Marshal Michael J.D. Walker, Baron Walker of Aldringham GCB CMG CBE DL was born on 7 July 1944, in Salisbury Southern Rhodesia, now Harare in Zimbabwe.

He was commissioned in 1966 and went on to serve in Cyprus, The Troubles in Northern Ireland and the first Gulf War in 1990/1991. He was also in command of NATO's Allied Rapid Reaction Corps which was deployed to the Balkans in 1995. He went to serve as Chief of the General Staff as well as the Chief of the Defence Staff. He retired in 2006 after having served in the British Army for a period of 40 years.

2011 – 2018: General Sir Charles Redmond Watt KCB KCVO CBE began his military career in 1972 when he was commissioned into the 1st Battalion, Welsh Guards. In 1982 he attended the British Army's Staff College at Camberley and later completed the Higher Command and Staff Course. He was promoted to the rank of lieutenant colonel on 30 June 1988, when he was just 38 years of age, and just two years later he was appointed as the Commanding Officer of the 1st Battalion, Welsh Guards. Further promotions followed, and on 17 August 1998 he reached the rank of major general and was made the General Officer Commanding, 1st UK Armoured Division, that was deployed to Bosnia.

By 2000 he was General Officer Commanding the London District. When the Queen Mother sadly passed away in 2002, Major General Watt, played a major part in her funeral arrangements. In 2005 he became the General Officer Commanding British troops in Northern Ireland. He retired in 2008 after having served in the British Army for 36 years.

In 1996 he was made an Officer of the Order of the British Empire (OBE). In 2004 he was made a Knight Commander of the Royal Victorian Order, and in 2008, a Knight Commander of the Order of the Bath.

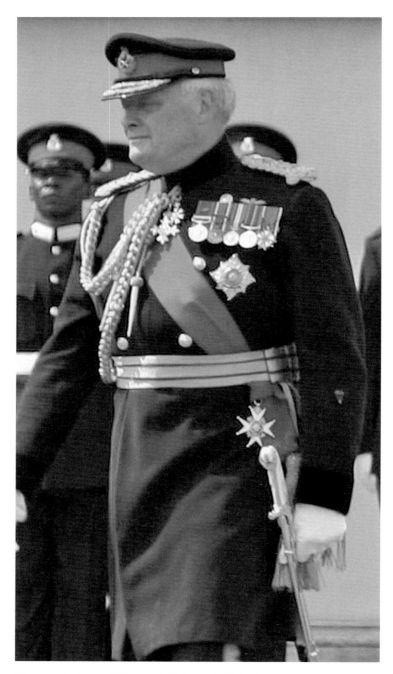

Figure 42: General The Lord Walker of Aldringham.

He is yet another man who brought with him to the role of Governor of Royal Hospital Chelsea, a significant wealth of military experience. He retired in September 2018.

When looking at the list of men who have served as the Governor of the Royal Hospital Chelsea, one can't but fail to be impressed with their credentials, nearly all of them having experienced war at its worst.

Chapter 9

The First World War at the Hospital

Friday, 7 August 1914 saw an inquest take place at Chelsea Town Hall, where the Coroner, Mr Walter Schroder, and a jury, looked into the circumstances surrounding the death of William Harvey, an in-pensioner at the Royal Hospital Chelsea, who died with tragic suddenness on the evening of Monday, 3 August 1914.

It was down to Colour Sergeant Winterholder, of the Royal Hospital Chelsea, to provide the formal evidence of identification and confirm that the deceased had formerly served in the 74th Highlanders Regiment. He had been an in-pensioner at the Royal Hospital since May 1912, and had enjoyed a period of sustained good health in the two years since, although when he first arrived at the hospital, he had been somewhat emaciated and in need of a good meal.

The Coroner: '*Was he a man of sober habits?*'

Colour Sergeant Winterholder: '*I could not call him a drunkard, but at times he took rather more than was good for him. Still, I never saw him incapacitated.*'

The Coroner: '*When did you last see him alive?*'

Colour Sergeant Winterholder: '*One day last week. He then seemed quite all right.*'

The Coroner: '*Did he ever tell you whether he had any relatives?*'

Colour Sergeant Winterholder: '*When he entered the hospital he said he had no relatives.*'

The Coroner: '*Was he friendly with everybody?*'

Colour Sergeant Winterholder: '*Yes, on the whole.*'

Private William Smith of the Coldstream Guards, who was stationed at nearby Chelsea Barracks, told the court that he did not know the deceased, William Harvey. His account was that about ten o'clock on the evening of 3 August, he was walking along Lower Sloane Street, heading towards Chelsea Barracks when he caught sight of the deceased on the opposite side of the road who appeared to be in some difficulty. He noticed that the man was holding on to the railings as he walked along and a short while later he sat down on the front steps of a house. Private Smith then crossed over the road to see if he could provide any assistance to the elderly gentleman and asked him where he had been. Mr Harvey's only reply was, 'I think I've been drugged.' Private Smith and another soldier then slowly carried Mr Harvey back to the Royal Hospital, where they handed him over to the duty sergeant.

The Coroner then asked Private Smith a couple of questions. *'Was the deceased injured in any way?'*

Private Smith: *'Not that I could see.'*

The Coroner: *'Was there any sign of a struggle?'*

Private Smith: *'No sir. All of the clothing was in order.'*

Police Constable John Henry Wilson, who was stationed at the Royal Hospital Chelsea, gave evidence to the effect that when he saw Mr Harvey on Sunday evening he was sober and appeared to be quite well. In fact, Police Constable Wilson could never remember a time when he had ever seen him in a drunken state, but on the night in question when he was brought back to the hospital, he described him as being 'insensible'. A doctor was then called but before he arrived Mr Harvey had passed away.

Lieutenant Colonel O.R.A. Julian, the medical officer at the Royal Hospital, told the inquest that since Mr Harvey had been an in-pensioner, he had not been medically treated for anything particularly serious and his death was totally unexpected. Lieutenant Colonel Julian had later carried out a post mortem examination on Mr Harvey and established that he was well nourished, that there were no signs of any violence and there was no evidence of the deceased having taken any poison. What had been noted was that Mr Harvey's heart was in a very poor state and was practically worn out, and that he would have been likely to have died at any moment.

Having listened to all the available information, the Coroner determined that Mr Harvey's death was due to heart failure following long-standing valvular disease of the heart. The jury returned a verdict of 'death from natural causes'.

On **Tuesday, 15 September 1914** an inquest took place at the Chelsea Guardians' Office in Kings road. The Coroner, Mr R.L. Guthrie, and a jury were inquiring into the circumstances surrounding the death of 70-year-old John Baker, an in-pensioner at the Royal Hospital Chelsea, who died in the hospital's Infirmary as the result of a fall in Sloane Square.

The deceased's son, William Baker, of 75 Haverhill Road, Balham, identified the body of his father, who had served in the British Army for 21 years in the Army Service Corps, and had seen active service in the Zulu War of 1879. Mr Baker had last seen his father alive on 30 July 1914 when, other than a cold, he appeared to be in good health. He had been shocked and surprised to hear that his father had passed away.

Colour Sergeant Wood of the Royal Hospital told the inquest that Mr Baker had been an in-pensioner at the Royal Hospital for nearly five years, and that during that time he had been in excellent health, although occasionally it wasn't unusual for him to drink a bit too much. Colour Sergeant Wood said that he had last seen Mr Baker alive at about half past seven on Friday evening, when he was leaving the Rose & Crown Public House, in Lower Sloane Street, at which time he appeared to be perfectly sober.

Police Constable 176B Wilcocks informed the Inquest that at about a quarter past eleven on Friday evening, he saw a large crowd gathered around the Sloane Square convenience. When he got to the front of the crowd he found Mr Baker sitting at the bottom of the steps and he appeared to be stunned. Police Constable Wilcocks tried speaking to him, but he made no reply, so the officer placed him on an ambulance cart and conveyed him to St George's Hospital. On arrival at the hospital Mr Baker was seen by Dr Ewart who noted a deep cut over his left eye. Mr Baker explained that he had slipped down the steps at the public convenience. None of the steps were dangerous in any way and there were hand rails on either side of the steps. Although he admitted to having had a little to drink, he was in a sober state of mind.

About one o'clock in the early hours of Saturday morning, Mr Baker was admitted to the Infirmary, where he was seen by the hospital's Medical Officer, Dr O.R.A. Julian, whom he told about having fallen over at the public convenience at the Sloane Square. He suddenly and without warning, became very agitated and excited, which resulted in Dr Julian having to ask him to calm down and remember that there were other patients in the Infirmary as well as himself.

About half past eight, the same morning as he had been admitted to the ward, he suddenly became unconscious and died shortly before midnight later that day. In the subsequent post mortem, Dr Julian noted the freshly stitched cut above his left eye. There was no damage to the skull, but there was evidence of a cerebral haemorrhage. Mr Baker had been suffering from Bright's disease which had probably made him prone to giddiness, and he had died as a result of a cerebral haemorrhage, no doubt brought about as a result of the fall.

The Coroner: *'Are Chelsea Pensioners allowed enough money to get drunk upon?'*

Dr Julian: *'Unfortunately, just now everybody wants to treat pensioners and soldiers. It is a bit hard on a pensioner who does not like to refuse a drink.'*

The Coroner returned a verdict of 'accidental death'.

On **Monday, 23 November 1914** an inquest took place at the Southwark Coroners Court. The coroner hearing the matter was Dr Waldo. One of the witnesses in the case was Joseph Goldsby, a veteran soldier who had served in the Indian Mutiny which took place between 10 May 1857 and 1 November 1858. The thrust of the inquest was to a certain degree taken over by the story which highlighted the sad plight of Mr Goldsby, who was surviving on 9d a day, and could not even afford to buy a solitary bloater (fish) which, he said, would have been a godsend.

The coroner said that owing to the publicity which Mr Goldsby's personal plight had attracted from a wider audience, he had received a number of letters from people who had sent in money for Mr Godsby which currently amounted to around £20, along with clothes and bloaters.

The coroner told the court that he had taken the liberty of interviewing Major Tudor Craig, secretary of the Veterans' Relief Fund, who stated that he was well acquainted with Goldsby, and would, with the veteran's written permission, act as his trustee, and secure him payment of 13 shillings per week.

Major General Sir Charles Crutchley, the Lieutenant Governor and Secretary of the Royal Hospital Chelsea, had written to say that Goldsby was formerly an in-pensioner at the Royal Hospital, but was obliged to leave because of his sickness at the time. He was then given a pension of ninepence a day. Goldsby had an excellent character and had served in the British Army from 1851 to 1861, the limited period for which he could enlist.

Goldsby expressed his gratitude and willingness to adopt Major Craig's kind suggestion, and the coroner arranged for him to go to the offices of the Veteran Relief Fund. A happy ending for all concerned, especially Joseph Goldsby.

On **Saturday, 5 December 1914** an Inquest took place at the offices of the Chelsea Guardians. The Coroner, Mr C. Luxmoore Drew and a selected jury, were tasked with examining the circumstances surrounding the death of William Welsh, who was 82 years of age, an in-pensioner at the Royal Hospital Chelsea, who had previously served with the 4th Hussars. He had died on the Hospital's Accident Ward on 2 December 1914.

An interesting aspect of inquests at the time, appears to be around the identification of the deceased because, despite being an in-pensioner at the time of his death and known by members of staff and fellow in-pensioners alike, a family member was still required to formally identify the body of William Welsh, which in this case was his daughter, Mrs Charlotte Penney, who lived at 25 Falmer Road, Walthamstow. She told the inquest that he was a man who enjoyed good health in a physical sense, but that 'he used to lose his memory at times and wander about not knowing where he was'. Today he would probably be classed as somebody who was suffering with either dementia or Alzheimer's Disease.

Eileen Cox, who was a masseuse nurse who worked at the Royal Hospital, gave evidence to the inquest that she saw William Welsh walking out of the ward when she was working on Ward 6 at just before seven o'clock on the evening of the day that he died.

The Coroner: *'Was he very much as usual?'*
Eileen Cox: *'Oh yes.'*
The Coroner: *'Did you tell anybody he had left the ward?'*
Eileen Cox: *'Just after seven when he did not return I informed the ward nurse.'*
The Coroner: *'Did you see him again?'*
Eileen Cox: *'No sir.'*
The Coroner: *'Was he friendly with everybody?'*
Eileen Cox: *'I think so.'*

William Stewart Towers was a Quartermaster Serjeant serving with the Royal Army Medical Corps, who was stationed at the Royal Hospital Chelsea. His main job was the dispensing of medicines. He told the inquest that he had known Mr Welsh for some eleven years and during that time he had never spoken about or intimated that he had thoughts of taking his own life.

The Coroner: *'Did you notice any changes in the man recently?'*

Towers: *'Only the senile changes, sir. He was bent.'*

The Coroner: *'What about his mental condition?'*

Towers: *'That was all right except for the fact that occasionally he used to lose his memory and wander about the grounds.'*

The Coroner: *'When did you last see him alive?'*

Towers: *'On Wednesday at 8.15. I was retiring to my quarters when an orderly came to me and said that Welsh could not be found. We searched and I eventually found him in the north compound of the hospital lying on the grass. He was groaning.'*

The Coroner: *'Did he say anything?*

Towers: *'All I could catch was "I'm ... Lavatory."'*

The Coroner: *'Would he have to pass the window that was just above him to get to the lavatory?'*

Towers: *'No sir, the window is in the lavatory.'*

The Coroner: *'How far is the lavatory from the ward?'*

Towers: *'The length of a passage. Fifteen to twenty yards, perhaps.'*

The Coroner: *'What is the window like?'*

Towers: *'Rather large and a sash window.'*

The Coroner: *'Is it kept open or closed?'*

Towers: *'Being a lavatory window, it depends upon whether anybody is in the room.'*

The Coroner: *'Did you examine the window when you had conveyed the man to the accident ward?'*

Towers: *'Yes. It was closed, and the blind was down.'*

The Coroner: *'The man was lying immediately below the window?'*

Towers: *'Yes sir.'*

The Coroner: *'Could he have been moved at all?'*

Towers: *'No sir.'*

The coroner appeared to be somewhat fixated on the lavatory window, the inference being that Mr Welsh had either climbed up to look out of the window at some passing troops, as suggested by the Coroner's Officer, Police Constable Pacey, and had then accidentally fallen through it, or had fallen from it on purpose in an attempt to commit suicide.

He was so fixated on the window in the lavatory that he called four more witnesses. Police Constable Pacey who examined the area immediately inside and outside the lavatory. Daisy Harwood, a ward maid, whom he questioned as to who could have closed the window. He recalled Eileen Cox, the masseuse nurse and asked her the same question and finally he called Dr Archer and he even asked him questions in relation to the lavatory.

Dr O.R. Archer was the medical officer at the Royal Hospital Chelsea and knew Mr Welsh fairly well. He said that his memory was defective and that he was prone to wander off around the hospital's grounds, sometimes late at night. Once when he was found at two o'clock in the morning, he said that he was looking for the toilet.

Dr Archer had seen Mr Welsh on three occasions on the date of his death: mid-morning, about 6.45pm and again at just after 9pm when he was in the accident ward, after he had been discovered in the hospital grounds. He went on to explain that he carried out a post mortem on Mr Welsh's body. He found a slight bruise above the left eyebrow, but there was no damage or fractures to the skull. The heart was in poor condition and heavier than was normal. The pelvis was fractured as was the lower part of the spine. There was a lot of internal haemorrhage and a fracture to the centre of the breastbone. Dr Archer determined that Mr Welsh had died of a heart attack caused by the haemorrhage and the shock of the subsequent fall.

The coroner didn't seem to comprehend the extreme difficulties and improbability involved in an 82-year-old man being able to climb 20ft up to where the sash window was, open it, climb through and jump or fall to the ground below. His implied suggestion that after Mr Welsh had fallen from the window, somebody then came along, closed the window, pulled the blinds down and then walked away, ignoring Mr Welsh, who one supposes would have been in some distress at this time, is, it must be said, risible.

There was also mention of another toilet, one that was for use by the nursing staff, which also had a window in it, but that was only about 3ft off the ground. Hardly a height for a fatal fall, even for an 82-year-old man, let alone result in a fractured pelvis and breastbone.

The outcome of the inquest was just as unusual. The coroner determined that there was insufficient evidence to establish whether Mr Welsh fell accidentally from the window or whether he committed suicide, despite the ambiguities mentioned above. In stating this he chose not to consider that a third party could have also been involved, which brought into question the possibility that he was unlawfully killed or even murdered, although the latter of the two outcomes is highly unlikely.

The coroner directed that the best course of action would be to return an open verdict, but despite this the jury decided on a verdict of 'Accidental death'.

1915

In **February 1915** the City of Westminster Council received a notification from the Commissioners of the Royal Hospital Chelsea, that there were vacancies for in-pensioners at the hospital and that in all probability, candidates who have been passed as eligible, would not have to wait more than one or two months if they applied immediately.

Sadly, a common theme about the stories that fill the pages of this particular chapter seem to include a large number of inquests relating to the deaths of Chelsea Pensioners, who were residents at the Royal Hospital, and who died in relation to falls, some of which were drink related in one way or another.

Friday, 16 April 1915 saw an inquest take place at the offices of the Chelsea Guardians in Kings Road, in connection with the death of 78-year-old in-pensioner, George Godfrey, who had died as the result of a fall in Radnor Street, Chelsea, on the evening of Monday, 12 April. Mr Godfrey was in the company of his son, who was a stoker in the Royal Navy. The question arose of whether the deceased and his son were drunk at the time of the fall. In fact, the son only managed to attend the inquest after he had appeared before the Westminster Police Court that very morning, having been charged with being drunk and disorderly.

As I have mentioned previously in this chapter there was at the time, what now seems the somewhat strange procedure of a member of the deceased's family being called to provide formal identification even when his identity was clearly known to others and not a cause of any debate. The death of Mr Godfrey had happened as a result of a fall he sustained whilst with his son, who was one of those in attendance at the inquest. But despite this Mr Godfrey's nephew, Mr William Morel, provided the inquest with evidence of identification.

Arthur Harwood, a costermonger, or what would today be referred to as street vendor, of 27 Smith Street, Chelsea, gave evidence to the inquest that on the evening of Monday, 12 April some time between eight and nine o'clock, he saw the deceased and a sailor, who were both strangers to him, standing at the corner of Radnor Street leaning against the railings. When questioned by the coroner, Mr Harwood stated that both of the men could hardly walk. They were leaning up against the railings and then the elder of the two fell to the ground and appeared to hit his head. Mr Harwood left his stall to assist the gentleman back to his feet and propped him up against the railings. The elderly gent thanked him for his assistance and Mr Harwood returned to his stall, only to turn round and see the man back down on the ground. By this time other people had gone to the elderly man's assistance and about half an hour later the Police arrived with an ambulance.

Mr Harwood confirmed to the coroner that Mr Godfrey appeared to be the worse for drink, and that besides not helping him the first time that he fell, the man who was with him in Naval uniform, was nowhere to be seen on the second occasion.

William Byrne, a corporal who was stationed at the Royal Hospital told the inquest that Mr Godfrey, whom he had known for about five years, was a healthy man, not a quarrelsome type, who like most men that he knew, liked the occasional drink. Corporal Byrne said that Mr Godfrey worked in the hospital's library and sometimes he would go out in the evenings, and when he did it was usually around about 8.30pm.

The Coroner: *'Would he have a pass to go out?'*
Corporal Byrne: *'No sir. He went out when he liked.'*

The Coroner: *'So it is not known when he left?'*
Corporal Byrne: *'No, sir, it is not.'*

Police Constable 661B Hearne who was stationed at Chelsea Police station, gave evidence to the inquest that about 8.15pm, on the evening of the night in question, he was on duty walking his beat when a member of the public approached him and said he was needed further down the street. As he arrived at Radnor Street he saw Mr Godfrey in the middle of a crowd being supported by two men, one on either side of him. He did not appear to be conscious and certainly could not speak.

Police Constable Hearne further stated that he noticed a wound on Mr Godfrey's head which was bleeding. He was carried down Radnor Street, on a hand stretcher by men of the Royal Army Medical Corps and was soon after met by a motorised ambulance which then took Mr Godfrey back to the Royal Hospital. Police Constable Hearne was able to establish from witnesses amongst the crowd that the injuries Mr Godfrey sustained came about as a result of a fall rather than a traffic accident.

PC Hearne also tried to speak to Mr Godfrey's son who he saw in Radnor Street, but he could not get any coherent answers from him as he was too intoxicated to speak, although he confirmed in response to a question asked by the coroner that the man had not been arrested and charged with drunkenness because he had not been disorderly.

Next to give evidence was James Godfrey, the deceased's son. He explained to the court that he was a stoker in the Royal Navy, stationed at the Royal Marine Barracks in Portsmouth, and had arrived in London on the Sunday to meet up with his father. He only had a short pass and had to catch the last train back to Portsmouth from Victoria railway station on the Monday evening, as he had to be back on duty first thing Tuesday morning. The pair had met at 11am on the Monday morning in the library at the Royal Hospital, where they spent most of the day. They left there at just after 6pm and went for a couple of drinks before making their way to Victoria station for him to catch his train to Portsmouth. He further stated that neither he nor his father were drunk, pointing out that because of his father's age he was unable to take more than a couple of drinks.

James Godfrey was asked by the Coroner if he and his father had at any stage leant up against any railings and he replied that they hadn't. His father's fall was due to him tripping whilst stepping off the pavement, and that he hadn't helped him back to his feet only because a crowd had quickly gathered around him which prevented him from doing so.

The Coroner asked him: '*What caused him to fall down?*'

James Godfrey repeated the question back to the coroner, in what could be interpreted as a faked surprised tone of voice. He followed that act of flippancy with. '*Now you want to ask me a question! I don't know, but I want to say it was not a submarine or a shell, or anything.*' His comments were not appreciated by the coroner, who certainly wasn't a man used to being spoken to in such a manner.

The Coroner: '*Nobody knocked him down?*'

James Godfrey: '*No sir.*'

The Coroner: '*He fell of his own accord, is that what you mean?*'

'*Yes, weakness and old age, I expect.*'

Prior to their meeting in London that day, the father and son hadn't seen or spoken to each other for more than ten years.

Lieutenant Colonel George Bray of the Royal Army Medical Corps, and the deputy surgeon at the Royal Hospital, told the inquest that he knew Mr Godfrey as he was the hospital's librarian. He was a reasonably fit man for his age and hadn't needed any medical attention for many years. When he was brought in on the Monday evening, he was unconscious. He quickly fell in to a coma,and died at two o'clock on the Wednesday morning.

A post mortem examination revealed that a fracture of the skull and a brain haemorrhage were the cause of Mr Godfrey's death, although there was no evidence of him having had a stroke. He also had three broken ribs, but this had not been part of the cause of Mr Godfrey's death.

In summing up and providing direction for the jury, the Coroner made the following comments. '*Of course if he was the worse for drink that would cause the fall. Do you want to say how the fall occurred? If you are satisfied from the evidence that the cause of the fall was drink, you must say so.*'

After the jury had deliberated over their decision for a period of time, Mr Drew, the foreman told the coroner, that they agreed with his decision of 'Accidental death' and decided to make no comment or observation concerning the issue of whether Mr Jacobs was worse for drink.

The sad thing about this particular case, is that it seems apparent that the deceased's son, James Godfrey, knew more about his father's death than he was letting on, especially in relation to the amount of drink that both of them had consumed.

Tuesday, 14 September 1915 saw an inquest take place at Westminster in relation to the death of Private Peter Lanaway, who was an in-pensioner at the Royal Hospital Chelsea, and who had previously served with the Grenadier Guards.

On the afternoon of Saturday, 11 September, Private Lanaway was seen to fall in to the River Thames at Chelsea. A local boatsman who was operating on the river close to where Lanaway fell in, managed to grab hold of him and keep his head above the water. But the weight of the pensioner's clothes, were made a great deal heavier because of the cold waters of the Thames, making it extremely difficult for the boatsman to continue holding him up. Fortunately, Mr W.H. Langley of the National Reserve was at hand. He dived into the River Thames and succeeded in not only holding up Mr Lanaway, but managed to get him into the boat allowing him to be taken to shore at Pimlico.

A verdict of 'found drowned' was returned, and Langley was highly commended for his bravery, the coroner saying that he would bring his name before the notice of the Carnegie Heroes' Fund and the Royal Humane Society.

1916

The week commencing **Monday, 24 January 1916** saw the Governor of the Royal Hospital Chelsea, General Sir Neville Lyttelton, attend the winter conference of the Charity Organisation and kindred societies at Denison House in London. The conference was looking at plans for the benefits of disabled soldiers and sailors. The governor told those attending the conference that of all the problems which had arisen from the war, there was none more pressing and important, and none to which the nation's people would demand with more insistency, an adequate and satisfactory solution, than that of the provision for disabled soldiers and sailors.

Up to that point in time, when the war was eighteen months old, it was estimated that between thirteen and fourteen thousand servicemen had been discharged from their individual branches of the military and absorbed back into the ordinary avenues of civilian industrial type work. With nobody at that time knowing with any degree of certainty how long the war would continue for, one thing was for sure and that was a much larger number of men would be discharged from the Army and Navy before it ended and not be able to return to their pre-war civilian occupation. In these circumstances the governor said, it was desirable, and would be extremely helpful, if charity workers and charitable organisations did their share in trying to resolve the problem, which before the war ended, would undoubtedly become a much bigger issue, the size of which could never truly have been predicted.

Wednesday, 7 June 1916 saw the St Luke's Mission Scouts inspected in the quadrangle of the Royal Hospital Chelsea, by its Governor General Sir Neville Lyttelton GCB.

No more fitting a background could have been chosen for such an auspicious occasion, than that afforded by the picturesque and historic buildings of the Royal Hospital, which for over 200 years had been a haven of peace, calm and tranquillity for war-weary soldiers who had given service to their country. Large crowds of interested spectators gathered in the quadrangle, many of whom were old, white-haired men who looked resplendent in their scarlet tunics, as they soaked up the spectacle of some of the nation's future soldiers lining up, waiting to be inspected.

At 8.30am Scoutmaster, the Reverend Capel C. Peacey led his group of enthusiastic and energetic young men into the quadrangle to the sound of bugles and drums, echoing around the Royal Hospital's buildings. They stood proudly to attention, before being inspected by Colonel E. Villiers, ADC, Scoutmaster Peacey, and General Sir Neville Lyttelton. After the inspection came the march past, with the salute being taken by General Lyttelton, who then gave his address.

He began his speech by making mention of the nation's feeling of great sorrow at the loss of Lord Kitchener, whom Sir Neville had the honour of serving under in two previous campaigns, and who was a person for whom he felt respect and admiration as an individual who possessed the quality of greatness. Lord Kitchener was, he said, a man who detested slackers of all kinds and he would be an extremely difficult person to replace, but he was also somebody who had set a great example to follow and a standard worth maintaining for future generations of soldiers.

Sir Neville had been more than happy to have been invited to take place in the Scout group's big day, for two reasons. Firstly, he had been friends with Colonel Villiers for more than fifty years and was extremely grateful for the work which some of these same scouts had undertaken within the hospital, as night watchmen, for nearly a year. They were also one of the finest Scout groups throughout the whole of London. They had won a shield for rifle shooting as well as placing teams in second and third positions at the recent National Rifle Association competition.

No doubt some of those Scouts would have been old enough to have enlisted in the Army before the war had ended.

On **Wednesday, 6 December 1916** the death occurred of 78-year-old Owen Broderick, an in-pensioner at the Royal Hospital Chelsea. The inquest took place on Monday, 11 December at the Guardians Office, the Coroner Mr C. Luxmoore Drew presiding.

Colour Sergeant W. Rowley who was stationed at the Royal Hospital, gave evidence to the inquest that Mr Broderick had been a pensioner at the hospital since 1911, having previously served with the 11th Regiment during his military service in the British Army.

On Monday, 4 December, Colour Sergeant Rowley was informed that Mr Broderick had taken a fall and was assisted to his bed by a fellow pensioner. Shortly after having been notified of this, he went to see Mr Broderick in his bunk and spoke with him about what had happened, and he said that he had fallen and broken his arm, but he did not say what had made him fall. Colour Sergeant Rowley immediately arranged for him to be taken to the infirmary.

Another in-pensioner, Charles Rolfe, whose bunk was near to Mr Broderick's told the inquest that he had heard him fall out of bed on Monday morning about five o'clock and went to his assistance. After helping to get him back in to his bunk he went and reported the matter to his superior officer. Another in-pensioner, George Hoddy, who was in the next bunk to

Mr Broderick, told how he heard him fall out of bed and call out for help. As he helped pull him up, he said that he had broken his arm.

Doctor Howard Coulthard, a Captain in the Royal Army Medical Corps, and who was stationed at the Royal Hospital, told the inquest that he had seen Mr Broderick in the infirmary on Monday, at which time he appeared to have fractured his left arm after he had accidentally fallen.

According to Doctor Coulthard, Mr Broderick died of general valvular disease of the heart, and was due to syncope, accelerated by the shock of the fall. After having heard all the evidence the jury returned a verdict of 'Accidental death'.

1917

On the morning of **Sunday, 17 June 1917** an inspection took place of some 700 members of the Corps of Commissioners at the Royal Hospital Chelsea, by General Sir Horace Smith-Dorrien. Whilst there he recognised and shook hands with several of the men who had served in various campaigns with him.

The Corps had been founded in 1859 by Captain Sir Edward Walter KCB,with the specific intention of providing work for ex-servicemen who were willing and able to work after the Crimean War, which makes it the oldest security company in the world. It is not just any old security company, because its head has always been the British Monarch.

The general had been among those who had for some years before the war, spoken about the inevitability of a European war coming about sooner or later, but even he hadn't contemplated that since the war had begun, some 24 million people from all round the world would be engaged in it.

In addressing those present, he said it was a pleasure and a privilege to him, an old soldier, to walk among the ranks of the Commissionaires, every one of whom had done something for the good of his country and the maintenance of the Empire. He thought it was a wonderful corps, quite possibly the best there was in the world. It owed its very existence to the affections of one man, for the benefit of old soldiers and sailors who had done their bit for the good of the country, and what he saw before him was a great tribute to Captain Sir Edward Walker's philanthropy, foresight and his power of organisation.

General Sir Horace Smith-Dorrien went on to say:

It must be a great satisfaction to you to know that of the 1,800 men of the Corps who have returned to the Colours, more than 100 have received commissions, a great number of decorations, and that two are commanding battalions.

What he failed to mention in his speech was of the 1,800 who had either enlisted or received commissions in the British Army, 150 of them had already been killed in action or died of their wounds.

General Smith-Dorrien had served in the British Army for forty-seven years, from the Zulu War of 1878–1879, where he was one of the very few British survivors of the Battle of Isandlwana, the Second Boer War of 1899–1902, as well as the First World War where he commanded II Corps in 1914. In April 1915 and he was sent home on the grounds of ill-health as he disagreed with the commander of the BEF, Field Marshal Sir John French.

An inquest took place on **Saturday, 18 August 1917** at Chelsea Town Hall, under the watchful eye of the Coroner, Mr C. Luxmoore Drew, concerning the death the previous day of 74-year-old John Hollingsworth, an in-pensioner at the Royal Hospital Chelsea.

Colour Sergeant John O'Brien from the Royal Hospital, was the person tasked with confirming the identity of the deceased, and he testified that he had known Mr Hollingsworth for just over two years and that he had previously served with the 18th Hussars. During his time as an in-pensioner at the Royal Hospital, he had been a patient in the infirmary on two occasions, although he couldn't recall for what ailments he had been treated. Mr Hollingsworth had very poor eyesight and wore glasses for everyday use as well as reading. As far as was known his only living relative was a cousin, Henry Wilmott, who worked at the Eastern Hotel, Limehouse.

Nurse Alberta Davies, who worked in the Infirmary at the Royal Hospital Chelsea, had seen Mr Hollingsworth the Saturday before his death on one of the wards, when he told her that he had been trying to cross the road in Piccadilly near the Ritz Hotel, thinking it was clear to do so when he had been knocked down, but he did not know who was to blame.

Police Constable 1000 Baker told the inquest that he had seen Mr Hollingsworth lying in the middle of the road and opposite the Ritz Hotel, he had been knocked down by a taxicab at 9.50pm on Saturday, 11 August. Police Constable Baker then conveyed Mr Hollingsworth by ambulance to the Royal Hospital and, although he was conscious, he did not say anything.

The driver of the taxi, Mr Walter Kendall, from Hammersmith, was later seen by Police Constable Baker. He told the officer that the man was in the middle of the road, and as he approached where he was standing, he stepped off the pavement area of the obelisk and into the road right in front of him, and despite shouting at him and sounding his horn, he struck the man. Mr Kendall stated that he was travelling at about six miles an hour at the time he struck Mr Hollingsworth. He explained that his taxi went over him, but not the wheels.

Mr Kendall in his evidence stated that there was a very dark night with no moon, but Police Constable Baker said that there was an electric standard (lamp post) where the accident occurred and quite good light for the time of day.

Sir Augustus Alexander Brook Pechell, a physician and surgeon from the Royal Hospital, told the inquest that he treated Mr Hollingsworth at about 10.30pm on the evening of Saturday, 11 August. On examining him he discovered that he was suffering with shock. There was a great deal of blood coming from a wound on his head, his upper left arm was broken as were four of his ribs, and there were severe injuries to his right thigh and hip, with numerous abrasions to his face and head.

Mr Hollinsworth died of his injuries on Friday, 17 August. A verdict of 'Accidental death' was returned by the jury.

1918

At the Westminster Police Court on **Saturday, 9 February 1918**, before Mr K.C. Francis, one case in particular caught the eye: that of Mr George Baker of 27 Jubilee Place, Chelsea, who was charged with begging at Elizabeth Street, Victoria, on the afternoon of Friday, 1 February.

Mr Baker, an Army pensioner wore campaign medals from his time in service, one relating to the march between Kabul to Kandahar, under General, later Lord, Roberts. In the spring of 1880, with a force of 10,000 men, General Roberts embarked on a legendary feat of British military history, when he marched from Kabul to Kandahar, a distance of some 300 miles, in just twenty days. In the brutal heat of an Afghanistan summer, the British managed to cover fifteen miles a day, which was a remarkable display of discipline, organization and leadership. On reaching Kandahar, General Roberts linked up with the troop's British garrison, and together they defeated the Afghan forces and brought an end to the Second Anglo-Afghan War.

Police Constable 214B Davies informed the court that he had seen Mr Baker begging from soldiers and after arresting him for that offence he found him to have thirty shillings in his possession, along with a Post Office savings book which showed that he had £130 in savings, which was a very large sum of money for the time.

Mr Baker had previously been an in-pensioner at the Royal Hospital Chelsea but was discharged from there for begging. The magistrate, Mr Francis, remarked that after having perused a report from the Royal Hospital, it transpired that Mr Baker was not entitled to wear the Kandahar medal, which he so readily displayed on his chest. He replied that it belonged to a relative, which still did not explain why he was wearing it.

In summing up, Mr Francis told George Baker that seeing as he had so much money at his disposal, it would be pointless dealing with him by way of a financial sanction, instead he sentenced him to a period of incarceration of one month.

In **May 1918** there was a very interesting announcement concerning the engagement of an extremely well-to-do couple. Miss Betty Spottiswoode, was the daughter of Mr and Mrs Hugh Spottiswoode, and the other, Lieutenant Gerald E.V. Crutchley, 1st Battalion, Scots Guards, was the only son of Major General Sir Charles and Lady Crutchley.

Sir Charles, was the Lieutenant Governor and Secretary of the Royal Hospital Chelsea between 12 February 1909 and 18 May 1918.

The slightly unusual aspect to this announcement was that Gerald Crutchley had been captured whilst involved in fighting in France, and held as a prisoner of war by the Germans since, 25 January 1915, some three years previously. He remained in captivity and wasn't repatriated back to England until 18 November 1918.

As of **Saturday, 29 June 1918** the following is a list of the items, along with the individual amounts per week that in-pensioners and staff at the Royal Hospital Chelsea, were allowed as part of the national rationing scheme.

Meat – 20oz
Bacon – 8oz
Fish (Fresh) or Poultry – 32oz
Fish (Preserved)
Bread – 98oz
Sugar – 8oz
Tea.
Margarine – 5oz
Suet.
Cheese – 4oz
Jam – 8oz
Rice – 4oz
Pulses – 4oz
Oatmeal – 4oz
Potatoes – 112oz
Fresh vegetables – 40oz

An interesting aspect of rationing was that different identified groups of people had different allowances. Fighting men would get more than say convicts and prisoners in civil prisons, but even within the different categories of hospitals the allowances were different. By way of example, pensioners and staff at the Royal Hospital had a higher weekly meat allowance than those in prison or interned aliens, but nearly half as much as those who were being treated in military hospitals.

On **Sunday, 8 September 1918** a film version of the Zulu Wars of 1879, entitled *The Symbol of Sacrifice* made by African Film Productions, was being shown at the Marlborough Picture Theatre throughout the course of the day, and at the London Pavilion, one of the more elegant theatres in the West End.

The Alhambra Theatre, which is situated on the east side of Leicester Square, in the heart of the West End, showed the film on Friday, 13 September, and what was particularly notable about this showing was that twenty-two in-pensioners from the Royal Hospital Chelsea, who were living veterans of that war, were in attendance to see the film representation of what they actually did at both Rourke's Drift and Ulundi. I do not believe it would have been possible to have twenty-two better film critics present at the showing of a movie as on this particular occasion.

Chapter 10

The Second World War at the Hospital

T he Royal Hospital Chelsea, its staff and the in-pensioners, were not exempt from the death and destruction of the war, in fact quite the opposite. The hospital was bombed on twenty-nine occasions during the war, with a total of 117 explosive or incendiary devices landing on its buildings or within its grounds. This resulted in twenty-one of its staff or in-pensioners being killed and a further thirty-three who were wounded.

The following is taken direct from the Royal Hospital Chelsea's War Diary:

3 September 1939 10.50 am. Church Parade as usual, only about six visitors being present. At about 11.30 am, as the Chaplain was finishing reading the epistle, air raid sirens sounded faintly in the distance. The Lt. Gov leant over and informed the Governor who immediately stood up in his pew and gave the order, 'March Out'. It was afterwards learnt that war had begun at 11.15 am.

The in-pensioners filed out of Chapel as usual, got their gas masks from their bunks and went to their allotted shelters. The signal 'Radius Passed', was sounded about 15 minutes later. Owing to a misunderstanding, the Hospital hooter was not sounded, but otherwise the pre-arranged procedure was carried out. It was discovered later that the alarm was a false one.

The alarm interrupted the wedding reception held by Captain Lockley to celebrate his marriage earlier that morning of his daughter, Joan, and Mr Davis. Mrs Lockley was away, having volunteered to assist in the evacuation of school children.

3pm, at an officer's conference at his house, the Lt. Governor authorised some additional precautions, including the making of a small sandbagged shelter at the foot of the East Wing main staircase to accommodate a few badly disabled In-pensioners.

6pm. The Lt. Governor authorised the Chelsea Gate Lodge being occupied by an auxiliary Fire Brigade's Detachment, who had arrived at his request about two days previously and were sleeping in the Chelsea Guard Room. The detachment, equipped with a trailer pump, towed by a taxi cab and consisting of a Sub Station Officer and seven men.

An actual hand-written account of the first day of the Second World War as it unfolded in the grounds of the Royal Hospital Chelsea – a truly remarkable and detailed record.

In **October 1939**, with the war just over a month old, a moving story of self denial by old soldiers who had long since retired from being fighting men, came from the hallowed corridors of the Royal Chelsea Hospital. A number of Chelsea Pensioners learned that Lady Knox, the wife of the hospital's Governor, Sir Harry Knox, was involved in a working party that made hospital supplies for the British Red Cross Society. They wanted to help the best way that they could.

Each of the pensioners received 3d each day, and as their request to help out was quiet and insistent, the Governor suggested that they contribute 1d a week, meaning that the monies raised each week would be in the region of 20s to 25s. This went a long way and was a great help towards the purchase of wool and other materials.

Despite the fact that it was the hospital's governor who had made the suggestion, it was evidently ignored by the pensioners, because at the time of their next pay day, a total of £2 14s was raised. In addition, some pensioners gave 10s notes, whilst others handed over their entirely weekly allowance of 1s 9d.

In reporting the matter to Lord Cromer, the Chairman of the Red Cross and St John War Association, General Sir Harry Knox, added that he was very proud of the unselfish attitude and commitment of his pensioners. Their sacrifice set a splendid example to all people of modest means. The wool purchased with the monies raised from the Chelsea Pensioners' donations, was then subsequently knitted into items by sixty pensioners who were residents at the Royal Cambridge Home for soldiers' widows at Kingston-upon-Thames.

In **February 1940** an announcement was made of the forthcoming wedding of widow, Mrs Sarah Ann Silvester and widower Mr Henry Lee, both of whom were 78 years of age. Mrs Silvester lived at Milmans Street in Chelsea, whilst Mr Lee had the prestigious nearby address of Royal Hospital Chelsea. He was at the time an in-pensioner at the hospital. This meant that the happy occasion of the couple's wedding, was tinged with an element of sadness for Mr Lee, as it meant that he had to give up his cherished position at the Royal Hospital, as its residents have to be single and have no dependents. No doubt that the new-found love of Mrs Silvester was more than a fair swap and in the circumstances, a more than adequate form of compensation.

The couple were married on 12 March 1940 at Chelsea Registry Office. They were driven to and from their wedding in a car that was decked out with blue, red and white ribbons, and on their arrival they were met by a large crowd that had gathered in expectation of their arrival. The new Mrs Lee, looked resplendent in a full length black coat and hat, whilst Mr Lee was wearing his ceremonial, Chelsea Pensioner uniform.

It was reported on **6 April 1940** that General Sir Felix Ready GBE KCB CSI CMG DSO who was Quartermaster General to the Armed Forces between 1931 and 1935, had died at his home in Kensington. He was 67 years of age.

He had a distinguished career having served during the Siege of Khartoum which lasted for ten months between 13 March 1884 and 26 January 1885, the Second Boer War between 1889 and 1902, and the First World War in Mesopotamia. He was also the General Officer Commanding Northern Ireland between 1926 and 1929, before holding the same position between 1929 and 1931 with the 1st Infantry Division based at Aldershot. He had also been the Colonel of the Royal Berkshire Regiment since 1930.

His military career had seen him decorated on six occasions as well as having been mentioned in despatches eleven times. He had also taken a keen interest in the Old Contemptibles' Association, of which he was president for several years.

General Sir Felix Ready's funeral service took place in the Wren Chapel at the Royal Hospital Chelsea on Wednesday, 17 April 1940. The Reverend H.T. Mahler CF, conducted the service, which was well attended by family and friends, along with dignitaries from the different branches of His Majesty's Armed Forces.

He was interred later the same day at Putney Cemetery, with the Royal Berkshire's Drum and Fife Band playing. The Berkshire Regiment also provided personnel for the firing party.

Advertisements in newspapers and other publications were placed throughout **May 1940**, by the Commissioners of the Royal Hospital Chelsea, announcing the fact that they were looking to receive tenders to supply in-pensioners and staff with a list of food stuffs for a period of three months from 1 July 1940. The items in question were as follows: bread, flour, tea and coffee, potatoes, fresh vegetables and fruit, meat, groceries, bacon, butter, margarine, cheeses, eggs, jam, milk, fish, fowls and rabbits.

Completed tender forms, which were obtainable from the Secretary's office, had to be returned by post to the Secretary, Royal Hospital Chelsea, London, SW3, by 11am on Wednesday, 12 June 1940.

In **June 1940**, the then Governor of the Royal Hospital Chelsea, General Walter Braithwaite, along with Major the Hon. J.J. Astor, proprietor of *The Times* newspaper. Admiral of the Fleet Sir Henry Oliver, who had held nearly every post in the Royal Navy, and Air Vice Marshal C.A. Longcroft, one of the pioneers of the flying service, were joint signatories to an appeal on behalf of the National Association for Employment of Regular Sailors, Soldiers and Airmen.

The appeal highlighted the fact that as a result of the war there would be a large number of men, wounded whilst serving their country, but whose injuries, whilst preventing them from carrying out any further military service, would not prevent them from working in a civilian capacity, so that they could carry on working for their country's war effort. The Association hoped that businesses would be able to release some of their more able bodied staff to undertake more arduous work, which in turn would make their positions available for medically discharged men from the armed forces.

On **Thursday, 19 September 1940** at a meeting of the Commissioners of the Royal Hospital Chelsea Lord Croft, the Under Secretary of War, disclosed that a large number of incendiary bombs had fallen on the Royal Hospital. He paid tribute to the work of the staff and pensioners for the manner in which they had successfully extinguished the devices. He said that on another occasion there had been a heavy high explosive burst at the gateway, but the pensioners remained as unshaken as the famous old building. He had heard of pensioners of over 80 who were with difficulty restrained from attempting to assist in putting out fires and had to be ordered back to shelter. *'The conduct of the aged pensioners subjected to this bombardment,'* he said, *'has been worthy of the highest traditions of the Army and is an inspiration to all of their young comrades of the Army today and all their civilian neighbours.'*

On **Sunday, 22 September 1940**, an in-pensioner at the Royal Hospital Chelsea, Michael Piernan, aged 67, was killed when he fell 40ft from one of the hospital's windows. Mr Piernan's death was a sad and tragic accident. His family lived in Church Street, Sligo, Ireland.

Thursday, 3 October 1940 during a German air raid over London, one of the places that struck, intentionally or otherwise, was the Royal Hospital Chelsea. One bomb found its mark and pierced a wall of one of the hospital's buildings, crashed through the floor and also damaged the floor below as well.

Fortunately, the in-pensioners who occupied that particular building were in their well-planned shelters and no one was injured. There was, however, one individual, Private Rattray, late of the 24th Foot, who was left feeling outraged at the turn of events, as he along with other valetudinarians, had been evacuated from the hospital's infirmary prior to the attack. It is said that an oak tree should not be uprooted once it is fifty years old, and as Private Rattray had already passed his 100th birthday, he had perhaps earned the right to be indignant at the need to move him to safer climes, even if was for his own benefit.

Initially, it was not possible for the newspapers to publish the facts that the Royal Hospital had been attacked by the Luftwaffe, they were only given permission by the War Office to do so on Sunday, 3 November 1940, when the full story was released. This included the fact that it was a high-explosive bomb which struck the east wing of one of the main buildings, that housed 150 of the 500 pensioners who were resident at the hospital at that time. Thankfully when the bomb struck, all but six of them had taken cover in the hospital's underground shelters. Six of the pensioners, could not be moved quickly enough, instead they were 'sandbagged' into a 'cubby hole'. After the bomb had exploded, they were initially buried under the rubble, but they were not injured, and managed to extricate themselves from the ruins and came out unhurt. A fine oak staircase, which was part of the original building, was destroyed in the explosion.

On **Wednesday, 30 October 1940** an inquest took place at Hammersmith Coroners Court. It was in relation to the death of Timothy Downes, a 61-year-old in-pensioner at the Royal Hospital Chelsea.

On the evening of 20 October Mr Downes was walking along the Royal Hospital Road, immediately outside the hospital grounds, when he was run over by a bus, which resulted in his sustaining a fractured skull; he died almost immediately.

Colour Sergeant Alfred Crabbe, also of the Royal Hospital, gave evidence to the inquest that Mr Downes had been an in-pensioner for some two years and that he was in good health and a very active individual. Crabbe continued, that as far as he was aware Mr Downes was neither visually impaired or hard of hearing.

The Coroner, Mr Stafford, asked Colour Sergeant Crabbe if Mr Downes had permission to be out of the hospital grounds in the late evening. '*Yes. He was due back at midnight.*'

Police Constable 606B McKenning explained that at 9.20pm on that evening, he went to Royal Hospital Road in response to a phone call that had been received at Gerald Road Police station. The deceased had already been taken to the Royal Hospital before he arrived at the scene of the accident, and there was a stationary bus near to Ormonde Gate. The driver of the bus said to Police Constable McKenning, '*It was very dark when I suddenly saw a flash which appeared to be his cap peak. He was right on the bus before I had a chance to pull up. I did all I could to avoid him.*'

The coroner asked what the weather conditions were like that evening, Police Constable McKenning replied that it was quite misty, and already dark by that time of the year.

'*Other than the bus driver, were there any witnesses?*' the coroner enquired.

'*I was unable to find any,*' replied Police Constable McKenning.

The next witness was the pathologist, Dr Skene Keith, who carried out a post mortem examination of Mr Downes's body. He told the inquest that the only external injury was a small bruise on the deceased's right shin, but that he had three broken ribs on his right side and that there was a fracture to the skull.

The bus driver, Henry Charles Rayner of 2 Fircroft Rise, Hook, who was a competent driver and held a clean driving licence, was the next to give evidence. He explained that he was driving an emergency bus to Wimbledon, and that his speed was about 10 to 15 miles an hour. *'I had only the side lights on. It was dark and slightly misty, and so far as I could see, the road ahead was clear and the first thing I saw was a slight flash from my lights catching on the peak of the man's cap. I was actually on top of him. I braked hard, but he was too close to do anything else. I think he was struck by the wing. When I pulled up he was lying just in front of the bus.'*

Mr Rayner explained that there was nobody about and that as he was an emergency bus, he was carrying no passengers at the time of the accident.

In summing up the coroner said he was satisfied that the bus driver did all he could to avoid the deceased, Mr Downes. *'Every user of the road, including pedestrians, must take reasonable care. The deceased may or may not have seen the bus. It should have been visible to him, but the driver could not see him until he was almost on top of him.'*

A verdict of 'Accidental Death' was recorded. What wasn't made clear, was whether Mr Downes was in the road or on the footpath when he was struck by the bus.

On **Friday, 7 February 1941** a service took place at Fulham Baptist Church, Dawes Road, Fulham, conducted by the Reverend H.G. Doel. The hymns sung were, 'Abide with me' and 'Sleep on beloved'. The service was followed by an interment at Fulham Cemetery, of Mr Edwin Minns of 23 St Dionis Road, Parsons Green, or Rectory Road as it had been named previously.

A large number of friends, relatives and work colleagues attended both the church service and the interment, including members of staff and pensioners from the Royal Hospital Chelsea, where Mr Minns had worked for many years.

Mr Minns, who was 65 years of age, had a fatal collapse in Fulham High Street while on his way to work. He was a boiler-house stoker employed at

Hammersmith. A post mortem examination revealed that he had died as a result of heart disease, which meant there was no need for an inquest to take place.

Mr Minns was a veteran of the First World War. The British Army Medal Rolls Index Cards which cover that period, show an Edwin Minns, who first arrived in France on 12 November 1915, served as a Private (SS/20676) in the Army Service Corps. Sometime after that he was transferred to the Labour Corps as a Lance Corporal (306524) and he was demobbed and placed on the Army Reserve on 23 February 1919.

In **March 1941** in-pensioners at the Royal Hospital Chelsea were hard at it in the hospital's spacious grounds displaying a vigour and enthusiasm that was quite remarkable for men of their age. The oldest of them was in-pensioner Taley, formerly of the Rifle Brigade, who was 85 years of age. The 'foreman' was in-pensioner Thomas Salt, formerly of the 60th Rifles, who at 72 years of age, was a mere youngster by comparison.

Not content with just looking after their well-kept flower beds, which were and still are, the envy of many a gardener, they had taken to growing crops such as carrots, onions, and potatoes, along a large part of the hospital's south terrace. Even the greenhouses, previously the sole domain for fledgling flowers and plants, had been given over to growing lettuces, cucumbers and tomatoes. The need for more food to be grown by families, communities and organisations, had become an important factor in the war effort on the home front, from which nobody was exempt. A better organisation to fly the flag for such a scheme, would have been hard to find.

With the Blitz at its peak, the Luftwaffe carried out one of the largest air raids on London of the entire war on **16 April 1941**. An aerial mine landed in the road immediately outside the hospital's Soane Infirmary, what is today known as the Margaret Thatcher Infirmary, and took out the entire East Wing. Thirteen people were killed including eight Chelsea Pensioners and four nurses, whilst a further thirty-seven others were injured.

The following is a list of those men and women who were killed on that fateful night. All of them were subsequently buried at the Chelsea Metropolitan Borough Cemetery.

William Cameron was 73 years of age and a Chelsea Pensioner who had previously served with the 2nd Battalion, Life Guards. He was originally from Elgin in Scotland.

James Hutchins was 51 years of age and a wardmaster at the Royal Hospital Chelsea.

Samuel John Jackson was 79 years of age and a Chelsea Pensioner who had previously served with the Royal Dragoons.

Patrick Johnston was 67 years of age and a Chelsea Pensioner who had previously served as a sergeant with the Irish Guards.

Olive Evelyn Jones was 43 years of age and an Infirmary Nurse from Glamorgan in Wales.

William MacGovan was 85 years of age and a Chelsea Pensioner who had previously served with the Duke of Cornwall's Light Infantry. The Commonwealth War Graves Commission has the spelling of William's surname as McGovan, but it is definitely the same person.

Edith McMullen was 52 years of age and a Long Ward nursing sister, who was originally from Liverpool.

Elizabeth Lilian Fisher Nicholson was 53 years of age and a Long Ward Nursing Sister.

Samuel Pope was 81 years of age and a Chelsea Pensioner who had previously served with the Shropshire Light Infantry.

Henry Augustus Rattray was 101 years of age and a Chelsea Pensioner. He had served as a Sergeant Bandmaster with the 1st Battalion, 24th Regiment of Foot, between 1862 and 1868.

John Sullivan was 80 years of age and a Chelsea Pensioner who had carried out his military service with the South Wales Borderers.

Edith Taylor was 55 years of age and an Infirmary Nursing Sister, originally from Birkenhead, Cheshire.

William West was 81 years of age and a Chelsea Pensioner who had previously served with the Hampshire Regiment.

On **Monday, 28 April 1941** tragedy struck the family of Captain Geoffrey May MC, a Captain of Invalids at the Royal Hospital Chelsea between 1931 and 1956, when his 17-year-old son Oswald Peter Joseph May was killed in a train fire.

One of the coaches on an express train travelling from London to Newcastle, caught fire near Claypole, between Grantham and Newark in Lincolnshire. The coach in which the fire started, which was the second from last, had been reserved for sixty-four pupils from Ampleforth College, a Roman Catholic boarding school in York, who were returning after the Easter holidays. The fire appears to have been noticed when the train reached Claypole, at which time the train's emergency communication cord was pulled, causing it to slow, but it didn't come to a halt until it approached the signal box at Westborough. Before it came to a final stop, several of the boys managed to jump clear of the coach and the enveloping flames, which by then had spread forwards and backwards, engulfing the two adjoining coaches.

Initial reports spoke of six of the boys having perished in the flames, with a further seven having been injured.

The London & North Eastern Railway Company released an official communiqué at the time stating that the coach which caught fire was the one next to the rear brake van. The train in question was a relief to the daily 12.45pm express, their statement added, that the train was stopped and that every effort had been made by the crew to extinguish the fire, but the coach that was immediately in front and the break van behind it, quickly caught fire before the train could be uncoupled and cleared of the blazing coach. Doctors from Newark hospital were brought to the scene to treat the injured.

The subsequent inquest and enquiry into the tragedy, which resumed on Wednesday, 28 May 1941, determined that the cause of the fire was lighted matches, which some of the boys admitted they had been throwing around the carriage. In summing up and declaring a finding of 'Accidental Death', the Coroner, Mr Theodore Norton said: 'I have to come to the conclusion that the fire started as a result of matches used by the boys, and also as a result cigarette ends lying burning and possibly thrown about.'

He went on to say that the boys were all properly looked after by the master in charge, Father H. Dunstan Pozzi, and that he was free of all blame. How Mr Norton could make such a statement almost beggars belief. I would suggest that if the children under Father Pozzi's control were smoking and flicking lighted matches around the carriage, and he wasn't doing anything to prevent it, or didn't know it was taking place, how could Mr Norton's claim that he, Father Pozzi, was properly looking after them hold any credibility whatsoever?

Despite some of the surviving boys freely admitting that there had been smoking and the flicking of lighted matches taking place on the train amongst the boys, Mr Norton said that he was not prepared to find anything of a criminal nature against any of the boys and they were all exonerated. Mr Norton appeared to focus more on the issue of the connecting doors between the carriages, which at the time were referred to as communication doors. It was the railway company's instruction to its staff, that to prevent third class passengers going through into first class compartments, or other passengers going into reserved coaches, certain connecting doors between the carriages on the train were kept locked. Regardless of whether doors were locked or unlocked, this would not have prevented individuals from alighting via the doors of the carriages that they were in, and it seems unfair and unreasonable for a railway company to have to take into account the possibility that a fire might break out on one of their carriages due to lighted matches being thrown about indiscriminately.

Whether any of the families who lost sons or had sons injured in the tragedy, challenged the findings of the Coroner is not known.

Apart from Oswald May, the other boys who died in the blaze were: Jean Pierlot, aged 15, and his 17-year-old brother Louis who were the sons of Hubert Pierlot, the Belgian Prime Minister, who was at the time living in London, leading the Belgian Government in exile. A third son was one of those who was injured.

Also killed were Ian Claude Emmett of Moreton Morrell, Warwickshire, aged 13; Richard Kennelly of Worthing, Sussex, aged 18 and Winthrop Park Fullman of East Molesey, Surrey, aged 16.

The May family lived at East Court, Royal Hospital Chelsea, and had done so for a number of years. Their other son, Ralph, had not been on the train, however, he was injured on 3 January 1945, when a V2 rocket struck the hospital.

In early **May 1941** Sir Harry Knox, Governor of the Royal Hospital Chelsea sent a letter to the Mayor of Chelsea, Lady Clare Hartnall, JP. thanking her for the assistance that was afforded the hospital by the borough in the aftermath of the Luftwaffe's attack the previous month which had damaged the infirmary.

The stretcher parties, ambulances, rescue parties, and all your wardens were most helpful. Nothing could have exceeded their promptness and kindness. Thanks to their help we were able to very rapidly clear the patients from our infirmary, and I am glad to say that, except in two or three cases, all the old men so rescued, will, I trust, be none the worse for their terrible experience. Would you convey to all concerned my thanks and the thanks of all in the Royal Hospital.

On **Friday, 27 June 1941**, widower, Mr George Weldrake, 65 years of age and previously of 16 Rokeby Street, West Hartlepool, was admitted as an in-pensioner to the Royal Hospital Chelsea.

He originally served with the 3rd Durham Militia as a youth and joined the regular Army in July 1893 at the Strensall Camp in York, when he became a private in the 1st Battalion Durham Light Infantry, later in the 2nd Battalion. He went on to serve for ten years, before spending a further six years on the Army Reserve.

Mr Weldrake described some of his military service:

I served in the South African War and came through without a scratch. I served in the last war and volunteered when Kitchener was raising his armies. Again I came through all right. My luck holds good for I was bombed recently at a house where I was staying in the North-East, and once more I escaped with little hurt.

I was with the Royal West Kent Regiment in the last war and won the Military Medal in France. That was when I shot German officers, put two machine guns out of action, and got valuable information for the officer commanding my company. I was peppered with machine-gun fire, but came to no serious physical harm.

I was presented with the medal at the Guildhall, Hull, by Sir Joseph Rank, the then Lord Mayor of the city. After being demobbed I stayed in Hull, and only returned to my native town about four years ago. I was born in South Street, in the Old Town, and wanted to see what the old place looked like. I have been trying to do my bit in this war as a voluntary air raid warden.

Just the thought of becoming a Chelsea Pensioner made Mr Weldrake a very happy and proud man, especially as he knew it would reunite him with some former comrades as well as other men like him who had seen service in the African wars and the First World War. He said: *'I've never had a black mark against me in the Army and never been up before the CO for being drunk, or being dirty and untidy on parade. I feel sure I shall be happy for the rest of my days among the old sweats at Chelsea.'*

The British Army Rolls Index Cards for those who took part in the First World War, show a George Weldrake, who was a Private (201212) in the Royal West Kent Regiment who later transferred to the Labour Corps, where he became Private 471094. His home address was then 17 Seamer Court, Seamer Road, Scarborough.

The British Army Pension Records show that a George Weldrake enlisted in the Durham Light Infantry as Private 4978 on 15 July 1893 at Strensall, when he had just turned 18. His subsequent service was in India for nearly five years between 1895 and 1900, and in South Africa between 1901 and 1902. Prior to enlisting in the Regular Army, he had served with the 3ʳᵈ Durham Light Infantry Militia.

George married Annie Shaw on 7 September 1902 at St Stephen's Parish Church, Hull. They went on to have three children. George, born in 1902, Elizabeth, born in 1904 and Lilian who was born in 1907.

He remained with the Durham Light Infantry until 20 December 1902, before being placed on the Army Reserve, where he remained until 14 July 1909, when he was discharged. Part of his Army Pension Record, also showed that he had re-enlisted in the Army Reserve on 6 April 1911 at Hull, when he became Private 5806 in the 3ʳᵈ Battalion East Yorkshire Regiment. He was discharged at Beverley on 5 August 1914 the day after the outbreak of war, the reason given was for having been convicted by the civil powers of a felony, but it did not specify the actual offence.

On 5 October 1914 he travelled to West Hartlepool and enlisted as a private (20517) in the 13ᵗʰ Battalion, Durham Light Infantry. In relation to question number eleven on his attestation form, which asked had he ever previously served in any branch of the military, he answered, 'No'. To question number twelve which asked had he truly stated in its entirety, his previous military service, he answered, 'Yes'.

He was appointed to the rank of lance corporal on 15 October 1914 and promoted to the rank of corporal on 29 January 1915, but then two months later on 17 March 1915 he was officially reported as being 'absent' and didn't return to his battalion until 26 March 1915.

There then followed an extraordinary turn of events. On 19 July 1915 George Weldrake deserted from the Durham Light Infantry, but just twenty-two days later on 10 August 1915 at Tonbridge, Kent, he fraudulently enlisted in the 4th/4th Battalion, Royal West Kent Regiment, which was a Territorial unit, using the name of George Wilson. His attestation form clearly states that it was an alias for George Weldrake, although this could have been added at a later time. His previous military service was recorded as the period from 1895 to 1902, even though he had enlisted in the Durham Light Infantry in 1893. It also did not include his time spent on the Army Reserve, which in the circumstances, was understandable.

His record then shows that he was 'to be summarily dealt with by the Commanding Officer of the 4th/4th Battalion, Royal West Kent Regiment'. He was given 14 days detention which he served between 15 and 28 November 1915; he also had to forfeit pay.

On 5 July 1916 he was posted to serve as part of the Egyptian Expeditionary Force, when he sailed from Devonport arriving in Alexandria, Egypt two weeks later. Four days later he was admitted to the 17th General Hospital in Alexandria with what was diagnosed as cellulitis arm, which in laymen's terms, means pain or inflammation. He remained a patient there for six days. On 25 November 1916 he was treated at the 1st/1st Welsh Field Ambulance for general debility. His health worsened early the following year when he was admitted to the No.27 General Hospital and treated for sclerosis of the brain, and despite attempts to treat his condition, he was invalided back to England on HM Hospital Ship *Letitia*.

When he was fully recovered, George joined the British Expeditionary Force and was sent to France where he arrived on 27 July 1918. It was whilst serving there that his true identity came to light and he was given a new service number of 20293, and his surname was changed to Weldrake. It was soon after this, on 17 September 1918, that he was awarded his Military Medal. He remained in France until 22 January 1919.

On 5 November 1917 he was transferred to the Royal Defence Corps, where he served with 251, 255, and 300 Companies. On 6 April 1918 George was once again transferred, this time to the 4th Reserve Battalion, Royal West Kent Regiment, and at the same time he was arrested, tried and convicted by the civil powers, and sentenced to three months' imprisonment which he served at HM Prison Maidstone, between 29 April 1918 and 14 July 1918, having had fifteen days of his sentence remitted.

He was transferred to the Labour Corps on 30 December 1918, where he served with the 93rd Labour Company. He was posted to the 184th Labour Company on 8 January 1919, where he remained until, aged 44, he was finally discharged on 8 April 1919, under paragraph 392 (xxv) of King's Regulations, his service being no longer required. The final page of his record, although not totally legible, appears to show that he was looking to join the Royal Navy. Whether he actually did so, isn't clear.

George Weldrake wasn't quite the clean-cut individual he claimed to be. That being said, he was a man who quite clearly wanted to do his bit for king and country, and wasn't looking to get out of serving, he just seemed to go about it in a very strange way. That he was a brave man is not in doubt, his award of the Military Medal was proof enough of that.

On **Saturday, 28 June 1941** eight pensioners from the Royal Hospital Chelsea, with a combined 160 years of military service between them, attended a garden party given by the Member of Parliament for Exeter, Arthur Reed.

The be-medalled old soldiers, each had stirring tales of derring-do to tell from their military days, serving in far off exotic parts of the British Empire, such as Egypt and South Africa.

Corporal-Farrier Arnold, formerly of the Royal Horse Artillery, described his pride at having been given the opportunity to serve during the First World War, by which time he was far too old for active service on the battlefields of France and Belgium. Instead he was part of the Remount Department, which was the body responsible for the purchase and training of horses and mules for the British Army.

Sergeant Barr, formerly of the Royal Artillery, had a few notable stories to tell and Corporal Beckett, who was 79 years of age, made a delightful speech, thanking Mr and Mrs Reed for inviting them to the garden party, and the friendship and hospitality which had been shown to him and his colleagues by all of those present. All that was left was for the pensioners to make the long journey back to their home at the Royal Hospital.

On **Saturday, 2 August 1941** Alfred John Oakley, a 21-year-old labourer who lived in a three-bedroomed flat at 15 Eddiscombe Road, Fulham, appeared before Mr Powell, at Westminster Police Court, to answer an allegation of stealing a lamp shade and a bracket valued at 5s, the property of the Commissioners of the Royal Hospital Chelsea.

Police Constable 300B Anderson told the court that the previous

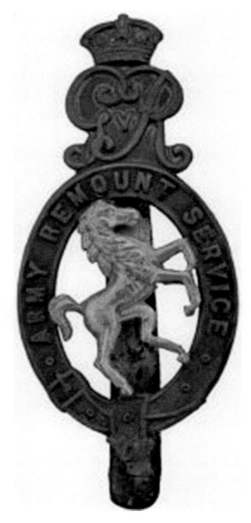

Figure 43: Army Remount Service Badge.

day, Friday, 1 August, he had stopped the defendant, Alfred John Oakley, and asked him what he had in a newspaper parcel on the front of his bicycle. Oakley admitted that it was a lamp shade and then produced from inside his jacket, a bracket and said that both items belonged to the Royal Hospital Chelsea, where he was working for an employee of a firm of contractors. His wages were £3 12s 6d a week, he was a married man who had been discharged from the British Army in October 1940 on medical grounds.

The probation officer told the court that Oakley had told him that he had seen the two items in question on a heap of debris and thought they were of no use to anybody. Oakley then told the court that he now realised the seriousness of stealing the property, to which the magistrate, Mr Powell replied by asking why he hadn't realised the seriousness of his actions before he had taken the two items. *'Have you got to be arrested before you realise what stealing means?'*

Oakley was fined 40 shillings for his misdemeanour, on asking for time to pay the fine, Mr Powell granted him a period of 14 days.

In **September 1941** Chelsea Pensioner and ex-bugler, Edwin Roger Delve, was in Bath for a couple of weeks visiting his sister who lived at 4 Caledonian Road, East Twerton. He had become somewhat of a celebrity in the city during his stay, as he spent most of his time proudly walking round the city in his bright scarlet tunic, peaked black cap, and a chest full of medals, which told the story of his life in the British Army. He had a smile and a wave of his walking stick for those who bid him good day and was more than happy to spend time chatting and explaining the significance of each of his medals. His new claim to fame was that he was the first Chelsea Pensioner to have visited the city of Bath. He had served in both the Second Boer War (1899-1902), where he faced near starvation at the Siege of Ladysmith, and the entirety of the First World War.

Friday, 3 October 1941 saw none other than 41-year-old Chaplain Arthur Ferdinand Gatehouse of the Royal Chelsea Hospital, brought before the Westminster Police Court to answer a charge of the theft of a dachshund bitch valued at £10, along with a leather dog collar valued at 1s. The prosecuting solicitor, Mr Claud Hornsby, told the court that he believed that the chaplain was a man of the highest character, and added, *'I think this matter might well be called, "Much ado about a dachshund."'*

The dachshund had been lost in the streets and taken to the local kennels, from where it was allowed to be taken away by Mr Gatehouse, who said that he would care for it until its rightful owner had been found or turned up at the kennels looking for it. He simply did not want it to be removed to the Police station or a dog's home. Mr Gatehouse had even taken the dachshund back to the kennels to see if the owner had been discovered or come forward. The more relevant question was how the matter had ever been brought before the court in the first place. Mr Gatehouse and his extremely prestigious address were well-known to the owners of the kennels, so there was never any uncertainty about who he was or where he lived, and at no time had Mr Gatehouse's *mens rea* been to steal the dachshund nor covet it as his own.

The case had originally begun at the same court on Saturday, 20 September and was adjourned before any evidence was heard.

Saturday, 4 October 1941 saw the death of 74-year-old Mr Joseph Merrigan, an in-pensioner at the Royal Hospital Chelsea, who was well-known to a number of MPs, as it was due to their efforts that he had been admitted to the hospital in the first place, his previous home having been at 5 Tonham Road, Thornton Heath.

He had been a patient at the Royal Hospital when it was bombed by the Luftwaffe, and was one of the thirty-nine patients rescued from the infirmary alive. From there he was transferred, along with a number of other patients, to Ascott House, Wing, Buckinghamshire, where he died a short time later. He was buried at Brookwood Cemetery in Surrey on Friday, 10 October.

An un-named official at the Royal Hospital said that there was little doubt that Mr Merrigan was who Bruce Bairnsfather, the First World War satirical artist, based his character 'Old Bill' upon. Not only did Mr Merrigan look exactly like the drawings of 'Old Bill' but he served in the same Warwickshire Regiment, and at the same time as Bruce Bairnsfather during the First World War. The only factor which gives any reason to doubt this supposition, is a statement attributed to Bruce Bairnsfather in which he stated that the character 'Old Bill' was a composite of numerous different individuals and was not based on any one.

Mr Merrigan was thought of by those who knew him as being a cheerful and popular individual, who took an active part in hospital life. There used to be a photograph of him hanging on the wall of the bar in the Coach and Horses Public House in Lower Sloane Street, Chelsea.

On **Wednesday, 19 November 1941** a number of cases were heard at Westminster Police Court before Mr Marshal one of which was in relation to Vincent S. Cassarley, aged 53 and a clerk at the Royal Hospital Chelsea. He was charged with being drunk in Royal Hospital Road. Police Constable Lee 346B told the court that he came across Mr Cassarley at 12.45am lying on the footpath in Royal Hospital Road.

The assistant gaoler added that Mr Cassarley had one previous conviction against him. Mr Cassarley admitted that he had been drinking liqueurs and that he wasn't used to them. He was found guilty and ordered to pay a fine of 10s. What, if any, action the Royal Hospital took against Mr Cassarley, is not known.

On **Saturday, 7 February 1942** the wedding took place at St Luke's Church in Chelsea, of Miss Mary Elizabeth Hobbs, who lived at 'Whitsters', Royal Hospital Chelsea, with her widowed mother, Mrs K.E. Hobbs, and Lance Bombardier Victor Henry Mills of the Royal Engineers.

The bride looked resplendent dressed in a traditional long white satin wedding dress and carrying a bouquet of carnations intertwined with heather and lilies of the valley. Miss Hobbs had two bridesmaids, who wore matching dresses of blue taffeta and carried bouquets of anemones. The ceremony was conducted by the Reverend Hogg of Newport, Isle of Wight, who had his own connection with the Royal Hospital Chelsea, having previously been one of its former padres.

Miss Hobbs was given away by a cousin of the bridegroom, and the best man was Mr Percy Mills, the bridegroom's brother. After the service a reception was held at the Royal Hospital which was attended by a large number of the happy couple's friends and relatives.

Before he enlisted in the Regular Army, the bridegroom had previously served in the Territorial Force, and prior to enlisting, he had been employed at the Acton Works of the London Passenger Transport Board. Miss Hobbs was employed as a clerk at the County Hall by London County Council.

Miss Hobbs' mother had lived at the Royal Hospital Chelsea for nearly 30 years, whilst her late husband Mr Hobbs, the bride's father, had been killed during the First World War.

A somewhat unusual letter appeared in a London newspaper **Friday, 13 March 1942** which had been sent in to the paper's editor by one of its readers:

Sir, Could you find a small place in your paper for this letter? I have been asked by the old soldiers at Chelsea Hospital if I could send them some cigarette papers and have done my best to obtain some, but have failed. I wonder if your readers would be kind enough to send some to No. 138 A.B. Everett, Ward 21, Royal Hospital Chelsea. I am sure someone will find a way. Thanking you, I remain, yours, etc.,

J.J. Martin, Ex-Sergeant
(Formerly) 1ˢᵗ Middlesex Regiment.

Monday, 23 March 1942 saw the tragic death of Second Lieutenant George Robert Edward Napier, of the King's Royal Rifle Corps, who died of his wounds at Wharncliffe Emergency Hospital, the day after having been shot during a field firing exercise in the Sheffield area. He was 21 years of age.

Lieutenant Napier was the grandson of Field Marshal Lord Napier of Magdala and Field Marshal Sir George White VC, the hero of Ladysmith during the Second Boer War, who was the Governor of the Royal Hospital Chelsea between 1905 and 1912.

The inquest into Lieutenant Napier's death took place in Sheffield on Wednesday, 25 March. Sergeant Basil William Hickman gave evidence that he was in charge of a section of nine men and was crouching behind a wall controlling the fire of a Bren gun. Lieutenant Napier was standing a little in front of him and to his right, in the role of umpire. It was his job to point out the position of the enemy that were represented by targets. There were also other sections at different locations firing at other targets with single shot rifles.

Sergeant Hickman said: *'I heard two rifle shots come very near to where he and Lieutenant Napier were stood, and made a remark to that effect to the deceased. A few seconds later I heard a loud thud and looked round to see the lieutenant lying on the ground, and heard him say, "They've hit me."'*

The men taking part in the exercise were all experienced soldiers and had considerable experience in the use of their firearms.

The medical evidence showed that death had occurred due to a haemorrhage caused by a bullet that had passed through the chest cavity from left to right. The coroner reached a verdict of 'Death from a gunshot wound accidentally received'.

The funeral took place the following day at Golders Green Cemetery. Besides a large number of friends and family being in attendance, some sixty members of his regiment were also present.

Monday, 25 May 1942 saw royalty at the Royal Hospital, in the shape of King George VI and Queen Elizabeth, who were guests of the hospital for the Founders' Day, or Oak Apple celebrations as it was also known. It wasn't the first time they had officially visited the hospital, but on the previous occasion they were the Duke and Duchess of York. They were received by the hospital's Governor and his wife, Sir Harry and Lady Knox, in their apartments.

The good weather allowed for most of the day's proceedings to take place out of doors on the spacious lawns immediately outside in the Figure Court. The Chelsea Pensioners, looking resplendent in their scarlet tunics with their shiny brass buttons polished to perfection in honour of the occasion, lined up on either side of the entrance way to the Great Hall and the Wren Chapel. Guests included the Mayor and Mayoress of Chelsea, Councillor and Mrs R.G. Wharam.

The hospital's in-pensioners and staff were all wearing a sprig of oak leaves in commemoration of Oak Apple day, which celebrates King Charles II's escape from the Army of Oliver Cromwell after his defeat at the Battle of Worcester on 3 September 1651.

Although the Royal Hospital Chelsea is for retired soldiers, all members of the armed forces were represented, as well as small contingents from the local Chelsea Civil Defence Service, and the Women's Volunteer Service, to commemorate the special occasion. As the royal party entered the Figure Court, the Royal Standard was unfurled by two Royal Navy ratings.

There were some 500 Chelsea Pensioners present that day, with their average age being 72. One of the oldest, Corporal R. McIlheron, formerly of the Queen's Bays, presented a bouquet to the queen. The king, accompanied by Sir Harry Knox, and the queen by Major General Morgan Owen, the hospital's lieutenant governor, carried out an inspection of the pensioners while a military band played. The royal couple spoke to many of the men and were keenly interested in the medals that adorned their chests, each one having a story as to what they were presented for. The more infirm pensioners were allowed to remain seated during the inspection, with the royal couple making a point of speaking to each of them.

After the inspection the king and queen mounted the specially erected rostrum, where His Majesty took the salute as the veterans of past wars marched by with a lightness of step that would have done credit to men many years younger. With the march past completed, everybody returned to their seats, and the king made his speech:

> *I am glad to be able to visit you on the 250th anniversary of the opening of the Royal Hospital, and I congratulate you on your fine soldierly appearance on parade. Your hospital has suffered from enemy action, but you are still proudly in occupation of these beautiful buildings, and your gallant behaviour under war conditions is worthy of the grand tradition of your regiments and of the standard which has been set by your predecessors here. You have helped in the war effort in every way which you have found possible, and by your good conduct and cheerful bearing in the streets of London you have set a fine example to everybody. I wish you all Godspeed and many peaceful years when victory is won.*

In response Sir Harry Knox, expressed his thanks for their attendance and kind words, and mentioned that for 250 years the hospital had been a home to the soldiers of the British Army. Most of the men on parade that day, he said, finished their active service during the reign of Queen Victoria. The men possessed many lovable qualities but none was more outstanding than that of their loyalty to the Crown, their Majesties had conferred a great honour in coming among them that day and the visit would forever remain a happy memory for all of those who were privileged to have been present. Sir Harry Knox finished his words of thanks with a call for three hearty cheers for the king and a special rousing cheer for Her Majesty.

Before leaving the Royal party visited the ruins of the hospital's Infirmary which had been destroyed in the air raid of 16 April 1941, which saw the deaths of thirteen people, eight of whom were Chelsea Pensioners.

Friday, 29 May 1942 was the 250th anniversary of the Royal Hospital Chelsea which was celebrated in style in the presence of a large gathering of invited guests. The occasion this year, understandably had a very special significance. King George VI addressed the Chelsea Pensioners who paraded at the Founders' Day ceremony which took place in the hospital grounds:

> *Your hospital has suffered from enemy action, but you are still proudly in occupation of these beautiful buildings, and your gallant behaviour under war conditions is worthy of the grand traditions of your regiments and of the standard which has been set by your predecessors here.*

Once again the late cool, spring weather allowed for a rain-free celebration, but one where the aged pensioners did not unduly suffer from any extreme heat in their thick, scarlet ceremonial tunics.

In the early hours of **Wednesday, 12 August 1942** Alfred Waters, a 74-year-old Chelsea Pensioner, died after he fell down some stone steps which led to a dug-out at the Royal Hospital. The inquest into his death took place on 20 August in Hammersmith. George Rossiter, who was employed as a storekeeper at the hospital, gave evidence that in the early hours of 12 August an alert was sounded warning of an impending air raid. He heard the sound of a loud thud and a short while later he found Mr Waters lying at the bottom of a flight of twelve stone steps, which lead down to a dug-out which was on the ground floor level of the hospital. He was bleeding from a head wound and was dressed in his blue coat and slippers and had apparently hurried to the dug-out when the alarm sounded. The assumption was that in the darkness, he had missed his footing and fallen down the steps.

Mr Waters died in hospital on 15 August, having never recovered consciousness. Dr S. Keith, the pathologist who had carried out the post mortem examination, determined that death had occurred as a result of concussion of the brain that was consequent with having fallen down the stone steps and struck his head. Having heard all the evidence, the coroner recorded a verdict that Mr Waters death was 'Accidental'.

The British Legion held a parade on **Sunday, 13 September 1942** at the Royal Hospital Chelsea. The salute was taken by Field Marshal Lord Milne, who was accompanied by General Sir Ian Hamilton, the Patron of the Metropolitan Area of the British Legion, and Admiral Sir Henry Bruce, who was the President of the Metropolitan Area.

The Governor of the Royal Hospital Chelsea, General Sir Harry Knox, was in command of the parade, which was attended by many of the Chelsea Pensioners. Addressing those on parade, Lord Milne said: *'We are going to face what will probably be the hardest year the world has ever known. We shall need grit and determination to see it through. It does not matter if we do not meet again next year, so long as England stands.'*

Steeped in centuries of history, the Royal Hospital Chelsea had become an iconic setting for such gatherings, as for many, just being at such a location was awe inspiring and morale boosting.

On **Tuesday, 17 November 1942** an in-pensioner from the Royal Hospital, John Walsh, aged 70, had a slight mishap when he fell down some steps at Victoria Railway station. In doing so he injured his left eye and side. An ambulance was called and when it arrived it took Mr Walsh to the Royal Hospital. He suffered no lasting effects and had fully recovered in a matter of weeks, showing to everybody the resilience of the Chelsea pensioners.

The death of Major Frederick Henry Bradley VC in Qwelo, Southern Rhodesia, was announced on **Wednesday, 10 March 1943**. He was 66 years of age. It was discovered in his will that since 1930, the £10 per annum annuity which he received as part of having been awarded his Victoria Cross, had been invested until ten years after his death, and that the proceeds which had been achieved at the end of that period, were to be given to the Royal Hospital for the benefit of the Chelsea Pensioners.

Major Bradley had been awarded his Victoria Cross when he was 24 years of age and a driver in the 69th Battery, Royal Field Artillery during the Second Boer War. His actions which won him the award took place at Itala, South Africa.

During the action at Itala, Zululand, on 26 September 1901, Major Chapman called for volunteers to carry ammunition up the hill; to do this a space of about 150 yards swept by a heavy cross fire had to be crossed. Driver Lancashire and Gunner Bull at once came forward and started, but halfway across Driver Lancashire fell wounded. Driver Bradley and Gunner Rabb without a moment's hesitation ran out and caught Driver Lancashire up, and Gunner Rabb carried him under cover, the ground being swept by bullets the whole time. Driver Bradley then, with the aid of Gunner Boddy, succeeded in getting the ammunition up the hill.

The full citation for Bradley's award, appeared in the *London Gazette* dated Friday, 27 December 1901. This also included notification that Gunner Rabb, Driver Lancashire, Gunner Boddy and Gunner Bull, were all awarded the Distinguished Conduct Medal, for their acts of bravery on 26 September 1901.

Saturday, 27 March 1943 saw the death of the Hon. Lady Lyttelton at St Mary's Convent, Chiswick. She was the widow of the Right Hon. Sir Neville Lyttelton, who was a former Governor of the Royal Hospital. The couple had married in 1893 and Lady Lyttelton accompanied her husband to many parts of the world, including South Africa. On a social level she did much to try and promote relations between the British and Boer leaders after peace between the two nations had come into being.

Sir Neville Lyttelton, who died in 1931, was the first Chief of the Imperial General Staff and became the Governor of the Royal Hospital Chelsea in 1912, a position he held for nineteen years until his death. Lady Lyttelton was by his side for the entire time in every sense, whilst dispensing warm-hearted hospitality to all those that she met. The couple had three daughters.

On **Wednesday, 14 April 1943** a porter who worked at the Royal Hospital Chelsea, appeared before Sir John Bertrand Watson, at Bow Street Police Court, in London, charged with being incapably drunk at Wilton Road, Pimlico, the previous afternoon. The man in question was 55-year-old John Baker. When asked by the clerk of the court if he wished to plead guilty or not guilty to the charge, Mr Baker replied that he was guilty of having had a drop too much. The court heard how, when interviewed about the offence at Gerald Road Police station, Baker denied the charge and a doctor had to be called out to examine him.

Baker had no previous convictions for any offence, including drunkenness, but he was still found guilty by the magistrate and ordered to pay a fine of 2s 6d and 7s 6d in costs, which was the doctor's fee.

Sir Bertrand was the Chief Metropolitan Magistrate as well as a Liberal Party politician. One of the most famous cases he was involved in, was the committal for trial for treason of William Joyce, also known as Lord Haw-Haw. During the Second World War Joyce made numerous radio broadcasts for the Nazi propaganda machine in an upper-class English accent which started off with the phrase *Germany calling, Germany calling*, although he was in fact an American of Irish ancestry. His broadcasts were put out by the Reich Ministry of Public Enlightenment and Propaganda with the intention of demoralising the troops and civilian populations of America, Australia, Britain and Canada.

Joyce was captured by the British Second Army on 28 May 1945 in Flensburg, northern Germany. He was tried at the Old Bailey and found guilty of treason and sentenced to death on 19 September 1945, although his defence team tried to have him acquitted on the grounds that he was an American as well as a naturalised German, arguing that Britain therefore had no jurisdiction in the matter. Sir Hartley Shawcross, who was the Attorney General at the time, successfully argued that Joyce's possession of a current British passport, even though he had lied to obtain it, meant that he had an allegiance to the king at the time he began working for Nazi Germany.

He was hanged at Wandsworth Prison by Albert Pierrepoint on 3 January 1946.

On **Saturday, 28 August 1943** the in-pensioners at the Royal Hospital Chelsea stood proudly on parade whilst they were inspected by Lieutenant General Jacob L. Devers, Commander of United States Forces in the European Theatre of Operations.

British veterans, most of whom had fought their wars before Lieutenant Colonel Devers was born, their hair grey and their bodies aged by many years of life, looked resplendent in their ceremonial scarlet tunics, adorned with shiny brass buttons and accompanied by their world-famous gold-braided, tricorne hats. With their campaign and gallantry medals proudly pinned to their chests, each of them looked as colourful as some of their military records no doubt were.

The American commander was visibly impressed with the pride and discipline displayed by the veteran British soldiers who stood before him, who were venerated as much that day as they were when their feats of soldiery were carried out years before.

Whilst the history of an old Dutch cannon was explained to their special guest by two of the Chelsea Pensioners, Private James Corbett, who was 77 years of age and joined the King's Shropshire Light Infantry in 1884, and Sergeant George Clarke, 71, who joined the Grenadier Guards in 1886, other pensioners took a keen interest in one of the Willys Jeeps which had brought Lieutenant General Devers and his party to the hospital.

One of the pensioners, Corporal David Williams, aged 76, who had enlisted in the 7th Hussars in 1889, seized the moment, got himself into one of the Jeeps and was taken for a spin around the grounds by American soldier, Private Albert Page from Shreveport, Louisiana.

After reviewing the pensioners, Lieutenant General Devers attended a service in the Hospital's Wren Chapel. He was accompanied by Major General Morgan Owen, the Lieutenant Governor of the Royal Hospital, Lieutenant Colonel John L. Campbell of the British Army and Major Robert Sevey of the US Army.

An inquest took place on **Thursday, 7 October 1943** at Hammersmith Coroner's Court, Mr Neville Stafford presiding. The case in question concerned the body of a newly born male child, that had been found in the grounds of the Royal Hospital Chelsea on Tuesday, 28 September.

Police Constable 447B Negus told the court that he found the body about 60 yards inside the hospital's grounds, wrapped up in a number of old newspapers. Dr C.K. Simpson, the pathologist who carried out the post mortem, gave evidence to the effect that he had been unable to establish any signs of the child's having achieved a separate existence, and that in all likelihood the child had come into the world prematurely and stillborn. There were no signs of any injuries. He was absolutely clear that he had found no evidence of any foul play involved in the death of the child. The coroner recorded the child's death as a stillbirth.

A meeting of the Chelsea Borough Council took place at the Town Hall, on **Wednesday, 27 October 1943**, which was presided over by the Mayor of Chelsea, Councillor R.G. Wharam JP.

During the course of the meeting the mayor announced that he had received a letter from General Sir Harry Knox, informing him that he had decided to relinquish the position of Governor of the Royal Hospital Chelsea. The governor wanted to thank everybody at the Town Hall for the continued assistance and support they had given to both him and the hospital during the five years he had been at the helm. He said: *'I leave Chelsea with the greatest regret and with many happy memories of the friends I leave behind.'*

The mayor said he was sure that they all regretted his departure. He felt that General Sir Harry Knox had done his very best to make the Royal Hospital a part of Chelsea. His one object had been to make the hospital a monument to Chelsea, not just another government building.

One of the councillors present, Mr Clapcott, proposed that a letter should be sent to General Sir Harry and Lady Knox, expressing the council's appreciation of their whole-hearted co-operation and the great interest they had taken in the life of Chelsea. It was a proposal that was passed and carried unanimously.

The new Governor of the Royal Hospital, the man chosen to take over from General Sir Harry Knox, was announced by the War Office on **Sunday, 31 October 1943**. It was General Sir Clive Liddell KCB CMG CBE DSO Reserve of Officers (Retired Pay), and Colonel of the Leicestershire Regiment. The appointment was with effect from Wednesday, 27 October 1943, the day that the previous incumbent General Sir Harry Knox, relinquished the appointment.

The new Governor's first official engagement was to inspect the parade at the British Legion's Remembrance Sunday parade and church service, which took place on the afternoon of Sunday, 7 November. The parade, which had a large turn out of spectators along the route, commenced from Manor Street, Chelsea, and was led by the band of No. 291 (Chelsea Squadron) Air Training Corps, followed by members of the Chelsea Branch of the British Legion. Others represented were the Chelsea Old Contemptibles, the 2nd County Home Guard, Chelsea Sea Cadets Corps, London Irish Rifles Cadet Corps, and the Chelsea Air Training Corps.

Before the service in St Luke's Church, a number of wreaths were laid at the Chelsea War Memorial, which is situated in Sloane Square. After the service the parade re-assembled before making its way back to Chelsea Town Hall, where the salute was taken by the Mayor of Chelsea, Councillor R.G. Wharam JP. Tea and biscuits were provided at the headquarters of the Chelsea Branch of the British Legion at 476 Kings Road, Chelsea.

There was an interesting case before the Edmonton County Court on **Friday, 11 February 1944** which resulted in the judge ordering a woman to return furniture valued at £1 15s to its rightful owner, a man by the name of Francis Kerslake.

Francis Kerslake was 87 years of age and a veteran soldier of The Buffs (East Kent Regiment), who had fought during the Zulu Wars of 1879. In 1941 he went to the Royal Hospital Chelsea for a visit to see if he would like to live there; he not only liked it, but he stayed and became a Chelsea Pensioner.

The furniture in question was what he had left with the woman for her to look after whilst he went to see if he liked the hospital or not. The un-named woman had interpreted this as Francis Kerslake giving her the furniture as a present and had refused to return it to him. What Francis did with his returned furniture is not exactly clear as he certainly wouldn't have sufficient room in his new home to accommodate it.

Josefa Reeve, a companion-maid who had been employed by Sir Clive Liddell and Lady Liddell for five years, had come with them when they arrived at the Royal Hospital for Sir Clive to take up his new position as governor. On **Tuesday, 21 March 1944**, she appeared at Marlborough Street Police Court charged with stealing articles worth £1 11s from a shop in Oxford Street, London. When she was arrested she had £14 in her possession and two post office savings bank books, showing a credit of £237. She was found guilty and fined 40 shillings.

Her counsel, Mr L.M. Minty described Mrs Reeve as the wife of a soldier who was serving overseas. He told the court that regardless of the outcome of the case, Lady Liddell had sufficient trust and confidence in her to take her back. Lady Liddell confirmed this statement to the court, saying that she trusted Mrs Reeve with her jewellery, some pieces of which were of great value. She had never at any point had the need to question Mrs Reeves or seen the slightest sign of dishonesty on her part.

Mr Sandbach, the magistrate stated that he saw Mrs Reeve's actions as an isolated incident, but he could not ignore her actions and fined her 40s, but with the amount of money she had in savings, she could comfortably afford it. The bigger question, which does not appear to have been explored any further, was how did a relatively low-paid maid manage to acquire the amount of money which she had in savings.

In **December 1944** Flying Officer/Navigator 160744 Douglas Frederick Haste of No.12 Squadron, the Royal Air Force Volunteer Reserve, who was 21 years of age and before the war lived at West Lodge, Royal Hospital Chelsea, was reported as missing in action, having not returned from operations over enemy territory. It was subsequently confirmed he had been killed in action when his aircraft, a Lancaster Bomber, was shot down over Germany on 29 November 1944. He was buried at the Reichswald Forest War Cemetery which is situated in the Nordrhein-Westfalen region of Germany.

On **Wednesday, 3 January 1945** Major 100465 William Napier of the Royal Army Medical Corps, died at the Royal Hospital Chelsea. He was 49 years of age.

He had enlisted in the Army during the First World War, whilst a medical student, and for a time he served with the Ulster Division in France, where he was mentioned in despatches. He resumed his medical studies in 1917 and went on to qualify as a doctor. In 1921 he became a Fellow of the College of Surgeons when he was living in Epsom, Surrey, quickly acquiring himself an extensive practice.

When the Second World War broke out he re-joined the Royal Army Medical Corps, and once again, for a time he served in France. On his return to England he was posted to the Royal Hospital Chelsea.

He was buried in the Ballee Church of Ireland churchyard, in County Down. Major Napier was survived by his wife, daughter, and son who was serving in the Royal Navy at the time of his father's death.

Mr John Ashton, who was 70 years of age and who lived at 83 Barracks Road, Hounslow, died on **Wednesday, 30 May 1945**. His Army Pension records show that he was a veteran soldier who enlisted in the Royal Fusiliers on 13 June 1896 at Aldershot, when he was 21 years of age, and went on to serve with them through a large period of the First World War, arriving in France on 16 November 1915. Before signing on with the Colours for a period of 12 years, I believe he had also served with their Territorial unit (4th Battalion) from as early as 1893, when he had reached 18 years of age.

After his initial attestation he was posted to the 2nd Battalion, who were at the time stationed in Belfast. He remained with them for nearly two years before he was posted to the regiment's 2nd Battalion on 2 February 1898. He was promoted to the rank of lance corporal on 14 April 1899 and further promoted to corporal on 2 August 1902. It would be a further four years before he was promoted to lance serjeant on 28 March 1906, and then just four months later on 27 July 1906, he was promoted to serjeant (L/5479).

He further served with the regiment's 6th, 7th, 22nd and depot battalions, before being transferred to the Labour Corps, also at the rank of Serjeant (356937), when he was stationed at Thetford on 30 August 1917, before he was discharged at the end of the war on 1 November 1918.

In the years immediately after the First World War, John Ashton was living at 54 Kings Terrace, George IVth Road, Hounslow, with his wife, Annie Sophia Ashton (née Groves), whom he married on 14 January 1907, at Brentford Register Office. They had three children, a son, John, and two daughters, Phoebe and Eileen.

Nine years of his 25-year military service was spent in India. He had worked at the Royal Hospital Chelsea for 22 years, as a messenger from 1923 until the time of his death.

Mr Ashton's funeral took place at Heston Churchyard after a service conducted by the Reverend G. Craggs. Floral tributes included those sent by the Old Pals of the 'Duke of York', and the officers and men of the Royal Fusiliers.

Sir Walter Braithwaite, who was the Governor of the Royal Hospital between 1931 and 1938, died at his home in Rotherwick on **7 September 1945**. He had served in the British Army since 1886. He saw action during the Second

Boer war of 1899–1902, and then the First World War as Commanding Officer of the 62nd (West Riding) Division, with which he was serving when the 8th Battalion, Leeds Rifles (who during the Second World War became the 66th Anti-Aircraft Battalion) were awarded the French *Croix de Guerre*. He was in charge of the 62nd Division from December 1916 until August 1918, and then only left because of his promotion to command the IX Army Corps, a position which he held until September 1919. He had led the division during the Battle of the Marne and in the victory at Cambrai. He was devastated by the death of his son on the first day of the Battle of the Somme on 1 July 1916.

The decision to make Sir Walter the Royal Hospital's Governor, was an excellent one, as he was seen as somebody who had the genuine interests of veteran soldiers, very much at heart. He also worked extremely hard for the Regular Forces Employment Association and pleaded its cause on one of his numerous visits to reunions in Leeds.

The second of the two wartime attacks on the hospital that resulted in multiple deaths took place on **3 January 1945**. One of Nazi Germany's dreaded V2 rockets, or the *Vergeltungswaffe*, the world's first long-range guided ballistic missile, scored a direct hit on the Royal Hospital, totally destroying the North East wing. A number of the hospital's other buildings were also damaged in the explosion. Some thirty-three of the hospital's staff and patients were injured in the attack, whilst five others were killed, all of whom were buried at the Chelsea Metropolitan Borough Cemetery. They were:

Major (100465) William Napier of the Royal Army Medical Corps, was a physician and a surgeon, stationed at the hospital. He had served during the First World War and had been mentioned in despatches.

His daughter **Deirdre Napier** was 17 years of age and a nurse working at the Royal Hospital Chelsea.

Camilla Margery May aged 47 years worked as a nurse for the Women's Volunteer Service, and was the wife of Captain Geoffrey Cruden May, of the Border Regiment, who was one of the Hospital's Captain's of Invalids.

Geoffrey Bailey was 63 years of age and held the position of Captain of Invalids at the Royal Hospital. He was the son of Colonel Christopher Bailey of Bushe, Timaru, New Zealand. His wife, Frances May Bailey, lived with him at the hospital.

Edward Joseph Gummer, aged 70, was a Chelsea Pensioner and the oldest of those who were killed. He was an Irishman, born in Dublin in 1874, who went on to serve in the 65th Regiment of Foot. He was the second of four brothers.

The memorial with their names displayed at the hospital includes the following words:

In memory of those officers, in-pensioners and residents of the Royal Hospital, named hereon who lost their lives within the precincts by enemy action in two wars.

It also includes the names of Ernest Ludlow MC, previously of the Grenadier Guards, who was a Captain of Invalids at the Hospital. His wife, Jessie, their two sons, Ernest and Bernard, along with their niece, Alice Copley, who were all killed during another air raid which took place on 16 February 1918, during the First World War.

Chapter 11

The Burial Ground Royal Hospital Chelsea

If you are visiting the Royal Hospital Chelsea from the direction of Sloane Square Underground Station, you would step out into Sloane Square and begin walking westward for about 100 yards, before turning left into Lower Sloane Street. Continue along the road until you pass Turks Row on your right-hand side. Although you are still in the same road, it then becomes Chelsea Bridge Road. Less than 200 yards later you come to a crossroads, where you turn right into Royal Hospital Road, and the hospital is immediately on your left. The entrance is further up the road, and walking towards it, you can see the hospital's burial ground through the railings. The first thing that struck me was how well it was kept. The lawns were immaculate and obviously tended on a regular basis. It was also apparent that all of the graves appeared to be very old, the dark grey colour of most of the headstones suggested that none of them were recent.

As you walk through the visitors' gate free of charge, greeted politely by one of the security staff, the cemetery is immediately to the left. There is a footpath which runs through the middle of the plot with most of the graves situated on the right-hand side and close to entrance and exit gate. Because of the age of some of the graves the inscriptions on some of them are not entirely legible; most are, although some are in Latin.

The cemetery has a number of graves and tombs dating back to the 1600s. There are also some fallen headstones that have been placed, as if they have been framed, on the wall that runs along the right-hand side of the cemetery as you enter through the main gate.

Both in the cemetery and also dotted around the hospital's grounds, there are a number of wooden park benches which have been donated by relatives of some of those who have been in-pensioners over the years. Where these individuals are buried, is unclear, but the names are included in this chapter.

Some of these men have extremely interesting stories, whilst for others, there is very little known about them. The following names are in no particular order, either alphabetically or date wise. It is more about where they are buried or located in the cemetery and the hospital's grounds.

At the far end of the cemetery, as it looks out on to Chelsea Bridge Road there is a tomb made out of Portland Stone, and although not all of the inscription is legible, some of it is. It is a family tomb for the Cheselden family and records the following names:

William Cheselden, died 1752.

Gulielmus Cheselden, died April 1752.

Deborah Cheselden

Gulielmi Cheselden, died aged 60, June 1754.

Gulielmi Deb Cheselden, died aged 17.

Wilma Deb Cotes

William Cheselden was the Royal Hospital's principal surgeon. He was both a surgeon and lecturer in anatomy and surgery and was one of those who was influential in helping to establish surgery as a scientific medical profession. He was admitted to the London Company of Barber Surgeons when he passed his medical examinations on 29 January 1711 at the age of just 23.

William Cheselden was an extremely intelligent man, who made some remarkable early breakthroughs in relation to certain medical procedures. In 1728 he was credited with carrying out an operation, the first of its kind, on a 13-year-old boy which helped him fully recover from blindness. When he was born

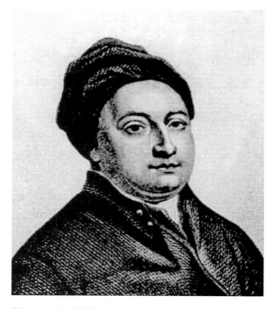

Figure 44: William Cheselden.

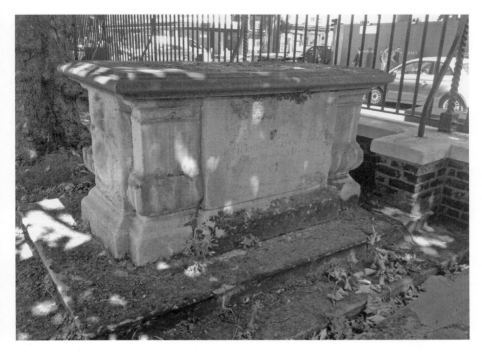

Figure 45: William Cheselden's Grave.

he had cataracts in both eyes, but after Cheselden removed the damaged lenses from his eyes, he was able to see again. Even today such an operation would require intricate, detailed surgery, yet this was an operation that Cheselden managed nearly 300 years ago. He was also responsible for coming up with a ground-breaking way to carry out the removal of bladder stones, a procedure which he first performed in 1728. He also managed to reduce the time that it took from hours to minutes, and with a greater chance of survival.

He died in Bath on 10 April 1752 at the age of 63, and is remembered as one of the true greats, and the forefather of modern surgery today.

Near to this is the single grave of **Kingsmill Eyre**, who died in 1743. We know that he was born in Newhouse, Wiltshire in 1682 and that his parents were Sir Samuel Ayers and Martha Ayers. I have not been able to establish the reason for the different spelling of the surname.

Kingsmill had three brothers, including Sir Robert Eyre, who was the Solicitor General 1708–1710 and then Chief Justice of the Common Pleas between 1725–1735, as well as two sisters. He was married twice, first to Mary Anne Eyre (née Lefever on 27 July 1721 at St Martin-in-the-Fields Church, Westminster. They had two daughters, Catherine, who was born on 18 April 1722, and Martha, who was born on 11 August 1723. Both were born at the 'Pensioners Army Hospital, Chelsea, London'. This indicates that they either lived nearby, or Kingsmill and Mary, lived on site at the hospital. Mary died on 7 January 1725, when she was just 25 years of age.

Kingsmill's second wife, Susanna Eyre (née Atkinson), was born in 1678 with whom he had three children. Sons Samuel, born in 1731, and Walpole, born in 1734, and a daughter, Elizabeth, although it is not known when she was born. Walpole and Elizabeth were both born at the 'Pensioners Army Hospital, Chelsea, London'. Susanna died in 1771, aged 93.

In 1716 Kingsmill was appointed as agent to the four Companies of Invalids at the Royal Hospital Chelsea, although at the time it was referred to as the 'Chelsea Hospital'. This was followed by his appointment as Secretary to the Commissioners of Chelsea College in 1718. He was elected as a Fellow of the Royal Society in May 1726.

There are suggestions that he was also involved in garden design and that he had also taken out a patent for a method of making iron in an air furnace using mineral coal, some time around 1736. At the time of his death in 1743, he was 61 years of age.

There is a headstone for a **John Newton** who died on 6 February 1788 aged 74 although it is not known what his connection to the hospital was.

Isaac Garnier died 1711. He is buried in an altar-shaped tomb, which contains a large inscription written in Latin.

Next to this tomb is a grave for **Daniel Garnier** who died on 26 April 1699, when he was just 32 years of age. The inscription on his grave is written in French.

D. Lefort died 2 April 1694. He was 39 years of age and left a wife, Marie Garnier and a 4-year-old son, Pierre Lefort.

Felix Cann died on 26 February 1786. The inscription on his gravestone says he was a Captain in his Majesty's Royal Hospital. Whether that means his rank in the Army had been that of a captain, or whether he was a captain of Invalids at the hospital, is not clear. At the time of his death, he was 86 years of age and more than likely to have been one of the in-pensioners.

John Murray died August 1775. He had been a sergeant in the Army and was about 75 years of age at the time of his death. He may also have been an in-pensioner at the hospital.

The next grave was interesting as it contained the bodies of not one, but three men. They are, **James Ford**, **William McMollon** and **James Gibson**. What makes it even more interesting is that they all died at different times.

The inscription for James Ford reads:

> *Here lyeth interd ye body of James Ford,*
> *Serjt. in ye Hon. Coll George Villerss Regiment of Foot*
> *in Cap Tho Ogles Comp. Pentio(ner) in his Majts Royal Hospital.*
> *He dyed ye 28th April Anno Dom 1698.*

The inscription for William McMollon reads:

> *Here lyeth interd ye body of William McMollon who departed this life ye*
> *20th Octbr. 1702 in ye 37th year of his age.*

The inscription for James Gibson reads:

> *This ston(e) belongeth now to James Gibson in ye 14 ward. Allso lyes ye*
> *body of James Gibson above said who dyed ye 17th of*
> *November 1714, aged 41 years.*

Besides the point of three men being buried in the same plot over a period of sixteen years, the latter two were relatively young to have been in-pensioners.

Captain Thomas Stuart was 82 years of age when he died on 26 October 1750. He was buried in a family tomb, which also included his wife and daughter, both of whom were called Ann.

He had been the Adjutant of the Royal Hospital for more than 30 years at the time of his death. His wife, Ann, was 89 years of age when she died, and their fourth daughter, Miss Ann Stuart, died on 11 November 1794 aged 58.

Another family grave has a father and son buried together, with thirteen years between their deaths. **William Barnes**, who was the son of Richard and Eliz Barnes, died 28 June 1786 aged 7. The inscription for his father reads: *'In memory of Mr Richard Barnes who departed this life April 18ᵗʰ 1799, aged 59.'*

Next is **Colonel John Campbell** who had held the position of Lieutenant Governor of the Royal Hospital Chelsea. He died on 18 April 1773.

The writing on **Nathaniel Smith**'s tomb is not totally legible. Next to his name it says *Major and Lieutenant-Governor.* That is then followed by *'Here lie buried the remains of Nathaniel Smith Esq, who died the 14ᵗʰ April 1773, in the year 7 of his life.'*

I could not find anything else to further explain who Nathaniel Smith was, and whether the above writings refer to a father and son of the above name. It would make sense that a child so young buried in the grounds of the hospital, was related to somebody who worked there of suitable high office.

The **Hon. Lieutenant Colonel Arthur Owen** had been the Governor of Pendennis Castle in Falmouth, Cornwall, which had previously been one of Henry VIII's coastal fortresses to help defend the nation against invasion by the French. He was the castle's governor for 21 years between 1753 and his death in 1774. Lieutenant-Colonel Owen had passed away on 17 October 1774 and was one of those buried in the Royal Hospital's cemetery. How he came to be buried there is unclear.

The next grave was sadly in a poor state of repair, and I could not make too much of it other than the name **Alexandri Inglis**. There is an inscription which appears to be in Latin, but it is hard to read as it is barely legible. The best I can make out is that he died in 1736.

Once again much of the inscription on this particular grave is weather worn and in a bad state of repair, but it is a family grave of the Pittone family. **Francis David Pittone**, appears to have worked at the Royal Hospital in some capacity, but I could not establish the date of his death. His wife, Sophia

Pittone, passed away on 22 June 1774. There is another female buried in the grave, Ann Pittone, possibly the couple's daughter, but once again what had been described about her age and date of death, had long since fallen victim to the ravages of time.

Theopelvs Cesill died 3 August 1695. His military rank was that of colonel.

John Ranby was a well-known surgeon of his time. He had started out as the apprentice to Edward Barnard, foreign brother of the Company of Barber-Surgeons, on 5 April 1715. His period of learning continued for more than seven years, before he was awarded the seal of the Barber Surgeons Company as a foreign brother on 5 October 1722.

He became a Fellow of the Royal Society on 30 November 1724, and first became part of the royal household's medical attendants in 1738. By 1740 he had become sergeant surgeon to King George II, before being promoted to the position of principal sergeant surgeon to the king in May 1743. As the king's surgeon he had to accompany him in the German campaign of that same year, and in this capacity he was present at the Battle of Dettingen on the 27 June of 1743. During the course of the battle one of his patients was the king's second son, Prince William, Duke of Cumberland, from whom he had to remove a musket ball from one of his legs. He managed to do so without having to amputate the leg.

In 1745 Ranby utilised his connections with both the king and certain members of the government, to have a Bill put through Parliament, which in essence was the forming of the body of surgeons, making it independent and entirely separate from that of the barbers. Ranby became the first master of the newly formed body of surgeons.

On 13 May 1952 he became the surgeon at the Royal Hospital Chelsea, taking over from William Cheselden, who had died and who is also buried in the hospital's cemetery.

John Ranby died on 28 August 1773 in his apartments at the Royal Hospital. He was 70 years of age. His death was somewhat sudden, as he was taken ill and within a few hours he was dead.

William Sparke's grave throws up the question of who else is buried with him, as the inscription on his grave includes: *'late Major to the 48*th *Reg of*

Foot and Major to this Hospital. Died 27th March 1775 aged 77, and others after 1800.'

Who these other people were, how many of them there are and why they were buried in Sparke's grave some twenty-five years after his death is unclear.

Another person buried in the cemetery is **David Crauford** who died in August 1723 aged 70. His role at the hospital had been that of lieutenant governor. Also buried in the same grave, is his wife, Catharine, but the date of her death and her age are not legible.

The Ogle tomb is interesting as it contains the remains of three people. **Sir Thomas Ogle**, the very first Governor of the Royal Hospital who was 84 years of age when he died on 23 November 1702. Sir Thomas's granddaughter, Harriot Cole, who was only two weeks old when she died, is buried with him, although the date of her death is not visible. The third person buried in the tomb is Utricia Ashley, who was the housekeeper at the hospital, aged 94 years when she died on 3 April 1749. It would appear that the tomb was erected at her request. How she was able to afford to pay for it is not known, as is the reason why she was buried alongside Sir Thomas, some forty-seven years after he died.

Mr and Mrs Grant are the occupants of the next grave. Mrs Mary Grant died on 21 December 1781. She was 56 years of age and the wife of Lewis Grant Esq who had been the Adjutant of the Royal Hospital Chelsea, for a period of thirty years leading up to his death on 16 October 1791 aged 75. Their daughters, Elizabeth and Mary Grant were also buried in the same plot, some time after 1800.

William and John Poulton are buried in the same plot, with William dying in 1705, and John in 1709. William, who in his life served four kings, died on 17 August 1705, when he was 79 years of age. John Poulton died on 19 March 1709, at the same age.

There is a small headstone with the name Mary **McIntoch** inscribed on it, who died on 1 September 1783, when she was 64 years of age. The inscription for her simply read: '*A loving wife and mother.'*

Colonel Thomas Chudleigh, a previous Lieutenant Governor of the Royal Hospital Chelsea, who died on 14 April 1726 when he was only 38 years of age, is also buried in the hospital cemetery.

The **Reverend William Keate,** the Rector of Laverton and the Prebendary of Wells in the county of Somerset, who died on 13 March 1795 aged 55 years, is another who is buried in the cemetery. The body of **Thomas Keate,** who was William's brother, was buried in the same grave. He died on 6 July 1821 when he was 76 years of age. Thomas was a surgeon at the hospital as well as being surgeon general to the Army and the king's surgeon.

The grave of **Captain Thomas Dawgs** also has the remains of his third wife, Ann Dawgs. He died on 15 January 1705 when he was 72 years of age. There are no further details concerning the death of his wife.

Elizabeth Symons was only 19 when she passed away on 12 January 1733. Her gravestone does not contain any other legible information about her.

William Lewis was 29 years of age when he died on 18 January 1706. He was one of the hospital's cook's.

The three children of Edward and Margaret **Sopps** are all buried together in one grave. Son Charles died in 1699, then Margaret in 1705 when she was three years old, and Mary, died the following year on 2 August 1706. It is not known how old she was.

Thomas Pond was another who worked at the hospital. By trade he was a carpenter, he died on 5 May 1731 when he was 63 years of age.

John Andrews worked at the hospital as a butler. He died on 29 March 1714 aged 66.

George Church died on 8 December 1792 at the age of 65. He was a controller in the hospital's coal yard, whilst also working as one of the porters. He had undertaken these roles for 34 years leading up to the time of his death.

Emanuel Langford was a chaplain at the Royal Hospital, who died sometime during 1724.

Alexander Reid worked at the hospital as a surgeon's mate. He died on 17 March 1715 at the age of 69. A surgeon's mate was a rank in the Royal Navy for somebody who was a medically trained assistant to the ship's surgeon. His duties were many including visiting patients in the sick bay, checking on their well–being, maintaining the surgical instruments, changing dressings on men's wounds and the administration of medicines, for which they were well paid.

Elizabeth Burney died on 20 October 1796 at the age of 68. **Charles Burney** presumably her husband, is buried in the same grave; he died in 1814.

Captain John Ramsey was 66 years of age when he died on 10 April 1696.

Colonel Thomas Dawson died on 4 April 1794 when he was 69 years of age. He had previously served with the Buffs or the 3rd Regiment of Foot. The inscription on his grave described him as follows: '*He was a most affectionate husband, a brave officer & a sincere & steady friend. In him the poor have lost a liberal benefactor & society a valuable member who was deservedly lamented.*'

Glowing praise indeed for a man who was obviously well thought of by all who knew him. Buried with him was his wife, Catherine Dawson, who had died nine years before her husband in 1785.

Another grave contained the remains of **William Daniel**, his wife, Mary and their niece, Mary Hill. William had worked at the hospital for thirty-one years leading up to his death, as the master cook. He had also been the master cook to King George II and whilst in that capacity he served the Duke of Marlborough whilst he was away fighting in his different campaigns. He had also served King William, Queen Mary and Queen Anne, and proved to be an excellent servant.

He died aged 75 years, but the inscription for the date of his death is sadly, illegible. His wife Mary, passed away on 1 August 1728 at the age of 55, and their niece, Mary Hill was just 31 years of age at the time of her death, the date of which is no longer legible.

Captain Walter **Compton**, died when he was 88 years of age.

I have written about **William Hiseland** in Chapter 5 and provided a full account of his extremely interesting life, so it only seems appropriate to take a look at what is written about him on his grave.

Here lies William Hiseland a vet(e)ran if ever (a) soldier was, who merited well a pension. If long service be a merit having served upwards of the days of man ancient but not superannuated, engaged in a series of wars, civil as well as foreign, yet not maimed or worn out by either. His complexion was fresh & florid, his health, hale and hearty, his memory exact, and ready in stature. He surpassed the prime of youth and what rendered his age, still more patriarchal, when above one hundred years old he took unto him a wife. Read fellow soldiers and reflect that there is a spiritual warfare as well as a warfare temporal. Born 6 August 1620. Died 7 February 1732.

The next grave contained the remains of six people. Husband and wife, Daniel and Eleanor **Jones** and their four children, Henry, Edward, Margaret and Elizabeth. Eleanor was the first to die on 9 July 1738, when she was 38 years of age, followed by Daniel, nine months later on 5 April 1739, aged 55 years of age. The inscription on the grave does not provide actual dates for the demise of the four children, just the ages for three of them. Henry was aged 4 years and 11 months, Edward was 3 months and Elizabeth was 3 years old. There was no age shown for Margaret, although it is believed that she was only a baby when she died.

Husband and wife **Richard and Grace Edge** are buried in the next grave. Richard is shown on his grave as being a *'Light Horseman in Chelsey Colledge'*. Richard died on 19 April 1724 at the age of 61, whilst Grace having passed away on 21 September 1722 at the age of 51.

Peter Warburton is shown as being a captain in his Majesty's Royal Hospital. Whether that refers to him being a Captain of Invalids, is not clear. He died on 6 June 1730 at the age of 94. His wife, Martha, followed him some seven years later, on 21 July 1737 at the age of 59.

Laughland and Mary Mackintosh have the bodies of their two young children buried in the cemetery. There is little information about them, other than their names were Laughland and Katherine Mackintosh, and that they died in 1714.

Captain John Bunting died sometime during the year 1732. Once again the ravages of time had resulted in much of the original inscription on his gravestone, becoming unreadable. He was 61 years of age at the time of his death.

Somewhat confusing are the two burials next to each other in the cemetery, with the same name. **Robert Rankin**. In one grave the man died on 12 March in either 1749 or 1750. In this case the man was 56 years of age. In the other grave, the Robert Rankin who is buried there, died on 13 January 1755. His age at the time of his death is not recorded.

Richard Johnson was 53 years of age when he died on Boxing Day 1734, that sadly, is all that is known about him.

A vault in the cemetery contains the bodies of four people covering a period of some thirty-six years. The first person whose remains were deposited in the vault were that of **Lady Renton**, the wife of Sir Thomas Renton who died on 11 June 1737. Sir Thomas Renton, who besides other well-deserved accolades, was also King George I's personal physician, died on 30 November 1740. In the same year, Mrs Margaret Nisbett, who was the wife of Dr David Nesbitt, and daughter of Sir Thomas Renton, died on 12 September 1740. She was 46 years of age at the time of her death. The last of the four individuals buried in this plot, is Dr David Nesbett, who died on 29 March 1773, aged 70.

Another grave with two people buried in it, is that of **Daniel Tiphane** and his grandson, **Stephen Liege**. Daniel was the wardrobe keeper at the hospital and died on 20 October 1750, aged 72. Master Stephen died on 25 July 1753, when he was just 9 years of age.

Mary Bettesworth was 47 years of age when she died on 8 June 1712, but it was another thirty-three years before her husband Major Richard Bettesworth joined her, when he passed away on Christmas Eve 1745 aged 88.

Alex and Mary Macdonald share the same grave in the Royal Hospital's cemetery. Mary died on 10 December 1772 at the age of 79, whilst Alex died fifteen years later on 21 November 1787, aged 87.

The headstone on the grave of **Simon Box** carries an extremely interesting inscription:

Here lyeth the body of Simon Box, who in the capacity of a soldier served King Charles the first, King Charles ye 2nd, King James ye 2nd, and their present Majesty's, King William and Queen Mary, whose pentioner he was belonging to this their Majesty's Royal Hospital and the first that was interred in this burying place, who deceased ye 6th of April in ye 63rd yeare of his age and of our Lord 1692.

There are a number of tombs and graves which are part of the cemetery at the Royal Hospital where the inscriptions have been eroded away over the centuries. These include two women who managed to pass themselves off as men and become soldiers, but there are no grave stones or tombs to mark their final resting place. Why this is the case is unclear, it simply appears that no markings were ever placed on their graves. The two women in question are Christina Davis who died in 1739 and Hannah Snell who died fifty-three years later in 1792.

There are others who might be buried in this cemetery including:

George Alexander and **Bert Kendall** are recorded on the same gravestone.

James Allen died on 13 November 1817. He was 48 years of age and a gardener at the Royal Hospital. His wife, Mary Allen, who died on 14 July 1826 at the age of 68, is buried in the same grave.

Frederick Walpole Anson was born in London on 21 May 1806 and died on 12 November 1848 at the age of 42. He was one of ten children of Sir George Anson, one of the hospital's governors. His gravestone says that he had served for more than 25 years '*after a zealous and most various service in India*'. He had been a major in the British Army. One of his four brothers had been a priest, the Reverend Thomas Auchild Anson.

Brigadier Frederick Lionel Banon was born on 2 June 1862, and died aged 90, on 23 August 1952. He was the commissioner of the Royal Hospital Chelsea for thirty years. Also buried in the same plot is **Ronald A. Banon** who was a captain in the 60th Rifles. He was born on 20 March 1893 and died on 23 August 1943.

Milbourne Bloome died on 8 August 1828 when he was 64 years of age. There are seven other people recorded as being buried in the same plot, they are: Mrs Mary Lucas who died on 27 June 1791, Sarah Lucas who died on 11 September 1796, Mrs Sarah Lucas who died on 22 September 1795, Benjamin Lucas who died on 11 March 1836, Elizabeth Lucas who died on 26 December 1826, Mrs Rebecca Bloome who died on 11 August 1852, Elizabeth Robertson who died on 26 December 1826, aged 76 and Christ. (an abbreviation for Christopher) Buckle who died 20 December 1660.

The inscription on **John Carley's** gravestone describes him as a '*Sixpennyman of this Hospital*'. He died on 13 July 1775. Also buried in the same plot is Mary Godd who died in 1780. Margaret Carley, John's wife, died in May 1785, aged 52.

Ann Cock died on 8 October 1826 when she was just 18 years of age. Buried with her is Frances Elizabeth Cock who died on 22 February 1810.

There are four members of the **Cooper** family all buried in the same plot. John Cooper was married to Maria who died on 23 February 1837 aged 67. Her daughter Maria Eliza Cooper died 4 June 1829, when she was only 13 months old. Another daughter, Mary Elizabeth Cooper died when she was 7 months old on 28 August 1835. Their son, John Cooper, died on 23 February 1836, when he was 7 years of age.

Anne Cossley who died on 25 October 1755, was the wife of Colonel John Cossley, who was the Lieutenant Governor of the Royal Hospital Chelsea. He died on 5 November 1765 and was buried alongside his wife.

The wife of Lieutenant Governor David **Crawford**, Catharine Crawford, died on 22 September 1713. Her husband was buried in the same grave ten years later in 1723. The actual date of his death has been eroded over time.

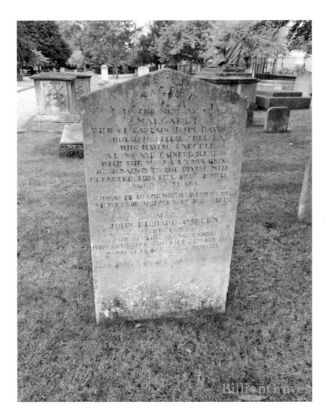

Figure 46: Davern Family Headstone.

The **Daverns** were next with three of the family being included in the same grave. The inscription on the gravestone reads:

> *To the Memory of Margaret Davern*
> *Wife of Captain John Davern*
> *Royal Hospital Chelsea,*
> *Who having endured*
> *A long and painful illness*
> *With the most uncomplaining*
> *Resignation to the divine will,*
> *Departed this life Feb 20th 1888*
> *Aged 30 years.*
> *Thanks be to God which giveth us the*
> *Victory through our Lord Jesus Christ.*

The inscription continued with Dr John Richard Davern:

Also John Richard Davern Surgeon, Son of the above named Who departed this life 25th Jan 1854 Aged 21 years and 8 months. Also James infant son of the above.

Major William Ebhart died on 31 January 1833, when he was 65 years of age. The grave also includes the major's grandson, Francis Knollis, who died on 10 April 1843, when he was only a child of 4 years and six months, as well as Major Ebhart's wife, Elizabeth, who died on 31 October 1835. William and Elizabeth Knollis, were married in 1811.

Thomas Edwards died on 4 March 1844 at the age of 63. During his life in the military Thomas was a private in the 2nd Regiment, Coldstream Guards.

There is a wooden bench in the grounds of the cemetery to the memory of **M.R. Esfandiary**, which carries the following, simple inscription. '*You are always in our hearts.*' He was born in 1934 and died in 2010. The surname has Iranian origins.

Sergeant Tom Fatimer doesn't have a grave in the cemetery, instead he has a park bench commemorating his name, with the following inscription: *'Donated by his family in loving memory of Sgt Tommy Fatimer 25.12.1908 – 4.3.2002, who loved these gardens. Grenadier Guards and in-pensioner of the Royal Hospital Chelsea.'*

Captain Thomas Gadsby, an in-pensioner at the Royal Hospital Chelsea, died on 19 January 1846 aged 71.

Hugh Percy de Bath Gleig was born on 20 June 1829 and died on 21 November 1845, making him only 16 years old at the time of his death.

General Sir Colin Halkett was born in 1774 and died in 1856. Unfortunately, much of the inscription on the side of his tomb is illegible, but it would appear that at some time during his military service, he had served in the Hampshire Regiment of Foot.

His was a military family. His father was Major General Frederick Godar Halkett and his younger brother was General Hugh Halkett. He had a distinguished military career which included the Peninsular War between 2 May 1808 and 17 April 1814. This saw the combined might of Bourbon Spain, the British Empire and the Kingdom of Portugal, pitted against the French Empire, Bonapartist Spain and the Duchy of Warsaw.

His military career had begun at 18 years of age, when he served with the Dutch Guards, where he remained for three years between 1792–1795, rising to the rank of captain. By 1 January 1812, he was the colonel commanding the 1st Brigade of the 7th Division at the Battle of Salamanca on 22 July 1812.

At the Battle of Waterloo on Sunday, 18 June 1815, he commanded the 5th Brigade of the 3rd Division. By the end of the day's fighting he had been wounded four times. It was a remarkable battle which saw the might of the French Empire, under the command of the charismatic, Napoleon Bonaparte, up against what was referred to as the Seventh Coalition, comprising the United Kingdom, The Netherlands, Prussia, Hanover, Nassau and Brunswick. It was a closely fought affair with either side coming close to winning the day, but the coalition under the command of the Duke of Wellington and Field Marshal Gebhard Leberecht von Blücher, finally secured a hard fought victory, with Wellington himself calling it, *'the nearest run thing you ever saw in your life'.*

The outcome of the Battle of Waterloo ended Napoleon's rule as the Emperor of France. On 7 July 1815 Wellington, Blücher and their victorious troops, entered Paris.

Colin Halkett became the Lieutenant Governor of Jersey in 1821. He went on to become the Commander-in-Chief of the Bombay Army in January 1832 whilst at the rank of lieutenant general. He became Governor of the Royal Hospital Chelsea in 1849, a position he held until his death in 1856.

Captain William Godfrey died on 26 April 1833, when he was 76 years of age.

Arthur Ronald Hutton was born in 1928 and died 2013. There is a wooden park bench which commemorates his memory with the following inscription: *'Arfer's Bench. In loving memory of Arthur Ronald Hutton 1928-2013 JP 1995-2013. Dearly missed by all. We'll meet again, don't know where don't know when.'*

John Hymes was born 1920 and died in 2013. A wooden bench in the hospital's grounds commemorates his name with the following inscription. *'In loving memory of John Hymes 1920 – 2013. Nothing loved is ever lost, and he was loved so much.'*

Stanley Denis Kennett, is another who has a wooden bench inscribed with his name in the grounds of the hospital. He is remembered with the following words: *'Sgt Stanley Denis Kennett 03/12/1925 – 27/03/08.'*

Colonel Henry Le Blanc died on 13 July 1855 at the age of 79. He had previously served with the 5th Veteran Battalion and the 71st Regiment.

The gravestone of **General Neville Gerald Lyttelton** informs any passing inquisitor that he is not buried in the cemetery, but that his ashes rest for evermore in its tranquil surroundings. It reads:

Here rest the Ashes of
Neville Gerald Lyttelton, General, PC, GC, BG, CVO
3rd son of George, 4th Lord Lyttelton of Hagley, Worcestershire.
Having served in the Army for 42 years in the Rifle Brigade, at the War
Office, and in High Command. He was for nineteen years the Governor of
this Hospital where he died on 16 July 1931 aged 85.
He was esteemed and beloved not only as a distinguished soldier and an
administrator, but as a Christian man, a leader, a friend,
and a great lover of English games.

Also, Katherine, his wife.
Daughter of the Rt Hon James Stuart Wortley. Born
18ᵗʰ September 1860, died 23ʳᵈ March 1943.
She took much from life and gave back to others abundantly.

The gravestone of **James McWarren** has not fared well over the course of nearly 200 years, with much of its inscription having fallen victim to the ravages of time. He passed away on 9 October 1835 aged 93. His wife Janet McWarren, is buried in the same grave, having died on 20 November 1835, just over a month after her husband. She was 92 years of age.

Dr Benjamin Moseley was a physician who worked at the Royal Hospital Chelsea. He died on 30 September 1819, aged 73. Also included on the headstone and buried in the same grave, is the name of William Henry Moseley, who died on 13 April 1827. Sadly, because of the erosion of the inscription, it is not clear what relation he was to Benjamin.

The inscription on the gravestone of **Archibold Parther** has become so badly eroded that there is sadly no more information available to mention of him.

John Fasson, an assistant secretary at the Royal Hospital Chelsea, died in 1848. Buried with him is his wife Frances who died 5 December 1869 aged 78.

Corporal Joseph Pearson who served with the Royal Regiment of Horse Guards Blue, died 11 February 1848 aged 59.

William Poulion died 17 August 1705 at the age of 79 and is one of those buried in the cemetery.

The gravestone of **Captain John Ramsey** simply reads: '*Here lyeth the body of Captain John Ramsey, who departed this life, ye 10 April 1696 in ye 66ᵗʰ year of his age.*'

Robert Rankin died on 13 January 1755 at the age of 25. His gravestone no longer is placed flush against one of the walls of the cemetery.

Sarah Ripley died 28 November 1834 at the age of 32. The rest of the inscription on her headstone is illegible.

The ashes of **Sir Dennis Thatcher** lie alongside those of his wife, immediately outside the hospital's Infirmary which is named after his wife, Baroness Margaret Thatcher.

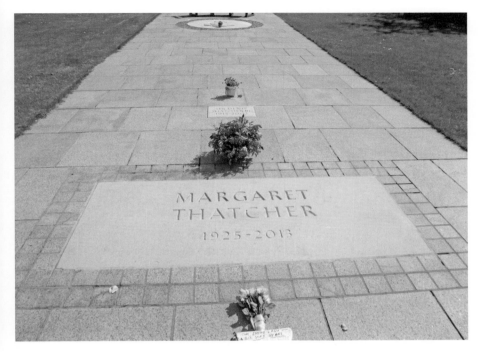

Figure 47: Baroness Margaret Thatcher's Grave.

Sir Dennis was born on 10 May 1915 and died on 26 June 2003 aged 88 years. Baroness Thatcher was born on 13 October 1925 and died on 8 April 2013 at the age of 87.

Gunner George A. Todd was born in 1907 and died in 2001. His name is commemorated on a park bench which is situated in the hospital's grounds.

John Vickers was an in-pensioner at the Royal Hospital, although his gravestone uses the older title of Chelsea College. He died on 1 January 1814 at the age of 72.

Benjamin Walker is buried along with his wife Elizabeth, but because the gravestone is in such a bad state of repair, it is not possible to determine any other information.

Captain Peter Warburton is buried in the cemetery but because if the condition of the headstone there is no more information about him.

George F. Whilds is another who is not buried in the cemetery at the Royal Hospital Chelsea, but who has a memorial wooden bench within the grounds. The inscription on the bench reads: *'Commander with the Duke of Wellington's Regiment, WWII.'*

Lieutenant Colonel George Williamson died on 6 September 1812 when he was 58 years of age and is buried in the cemetery at the Royal Hospital Chelsea. Colonel James Williamson died on 4 December 1813 aged 71. He was George's elder brother and is buried in the same grave.

Sam Wyatt was a London-based architect and clerk of the works at the Royal Hospital Chelsea. He was born in Staffordshire on 8 September 1737 and died on 8 February 1807, at 70 years of age.

James O'Hara, 2nd Baron Tyrawley and 1st Baron Kilmaine is buried, not in the cemetery but, in the Wren Chapel. Despite this honour I could find no obvious connection between him and the hospital, although there must have been one. He was born in Ireland in 1682 to Charles O'Hara, 1st Baron

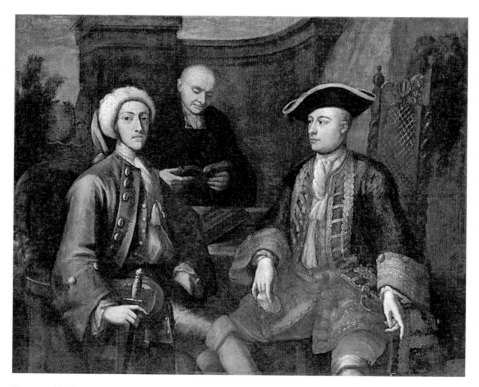

Figure 48: James O'Hara.

Tyrawley, and Frances O'Hara (née Rouse). He did not marry until he was 42 years of age, but with the life he had in the military up until that point, romance was quite possibly the last thing on his mind.

He was commissioned as a lieutenant in the Royal Fusiliers on 15 March 1703, and further promoted to captain two years later. He first saw action at the Siege of Barcelona in April 1706. He fought again at the Battle of Almansa in Spain during the War of the Spanish Succession, where he was wounded. The battle saw the combined Allied forces of England, Portugal and the United Provinces, soundly beaten by the armies of France and Bourbon Spain.

Whilst acting as aide-de-camp to the Duke of Marlborough he was wounded at the Battle of Malplaquet, France in September 1709. In January 1713 he succeeded his father as Colonel of the Royal Fusiliers and then spent a few years serving with them in Minorca, before becoming aide-de-camp to King George I in 1717. During his military career he was the colonel of seven other regiments, as well as being the Governor of Minorca, Gibraltar and Portsmouth.

He married Mary Stewart, the daughter of the 2nd Viscount Mountjoy, in November 1724. The couple had no children, although he did have at least two illegitimate children. His son Charles, followed him in to the Army, and his daughter, Georgina Bellamy, who was also known by the names George Anne Bellamy, became quite a well-known actress on the London stage.

James O'Hara died in Twickenham on 14 July 1774.

Chapter 12

Christian Davies and Hannah Snell

Christian Davies was born in Dublin in 1667 as Christian Cavanagh. Although her parents were Protestants, they supported King James II during his military campaign in Ireland, in what was known as the Williamite War between 12 March 1689 and 3 October 1691. Christian's father served in the Jacobite Army and died as a result of his wounds sustained during the fighting at the Battle of Aughrim on 12 July 1691. The battle was a bloody affair, with more than 7,000 men from both sides, either killed outright or, like Christian's father, who died soon afterwards from their wounds. By the close of the day, Jacobitism in Ireland was effectively at an end.

As a result of her parents' support of King James II and the Jacobite movement, the family's property was confiscated by order of William III, King of England, Scotland, and Ireland between 1689 until his death on 8 March 1702. Before the war Christian's father had been a local brewer.

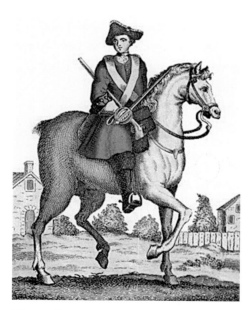

Figure 49: Christian Davies.

When exactly is not clear, but Christian left home and went to live in Dublin with her aunt who ran a pub. One of her aunt's servants, Richard Welsh, took a shine to her and soon they were married. When her aunt died, Christian inherited the pub, where she and Richard worked hard together to make the business work. Their marriage was blessed with two children and in 1691, whilst Christian was pregnant with a third child, Richard inexplicably disappeared one morning. He left without saying a word or providing any kind of explanation as to where he had gone.

It transpired that Richard had ended up in the British Army and was serving in Holland. Whether he had voluntarily enlisted or been press-ganged into joining the Army is not clear, but either way he was a soldier, which wasn't something he could do anything about in the short term. He couldn't just leave and return to his home and family unless he wished to be treated as a deserter. Richard had written a number of letters to Christian, explaining his circumstances but she never received them, but eventually one arrived at her home.

The arrival of this letter and her love for her husband would appear to be the reason behind her desire to become a soldier, rather than some misplaced desire to fight for her king and country. By joining the Army she hoped to get to where Richard was, regardless of whether they were in the same regiment or not. She left her children with her mother, cut her hair, dressed as a man and enlisted in Captain Tichborne's Company of Foot. Over the coming years she also used the name of Kit Cavanagh and later acquired the nickname Mother Ross, due to a brief relationship she had with a Captain Ross.

On 29 July 1693 she was involved in the Battle of Landen in present day Belgium. An Army from England, Scotland and the Dutch Republic, estimated to be in the region of 50,000 men, and under the command of King William III, took on a French Army commanded by the Duc de Luxembourg, which at 66,000 in strength, was slightly larger. By the end of the day the French had lost 8,000 men killed, with a further 1,000 who were either missing or captured. William III's Army suffered larger casualties, with 12,000 men who had been killed or wounded and a further 2,000 who were missing or had been captured.

Christian had been wounded during the fighting and taken prisoner by the French. She remained in captivity until the following year when she was returned to England as part of a prisoner exchange. If the French had discovered her secret, they certainly didn't let on about it when they returned her, which meant that the British authorities, still did not know her true identity.

Some time after her return, possibly in early 1697, and whilst still serving as a soldier in the British Army, she became possibly the only British woman to have taken part in a duel. Ironically, the dispute between Christian and a sergeant in the company in which she served, was over a woman. She won the duel, killing her opponent in the process. Soon afterwards she was discharged from the Army, whether as a direct result of the duel, is not clear, but what is clear is that it wasn't something she wanted to happen. No sooner had she been discharged than she re-enlisted in the 4th Royal North British Dragoons, which would later become the Scots Greys. In Christian's time, dragoons were mounted infantry who used their horses as transport to get them to different locations, but then dismounted to fight on foot.

She continued fighting up until the end of the Nine Years War, or what was also known as the War of the League of Augsburg. The end of the fighting, which resulted in her being demobilized, came about as due to the signing of the Treaty of Ryswick, now Rijswijk in Holland, which was signed on 20 September 1697.

Christian continued her search for her husband, despite not knowing if he was still a soldier, where he might be or even if he was still alive. With the beginning of the War of the Spanish Succession in 1701, she re-enlisted with what had now become the Scots Greys. Once again living a military life, although she worked, ate and slept next to her colleagues, nobody was any the wiser that she was a woman. The fact she had been able to keep her sexuality a secret for so long in such circumstances was truly remarkable. It is hard to comprehend that somebody wouldn't have picked up her lack of facial hair after a few days of fighting and without the opportunity to shave. The everyday function of having to go to the toilet with men standing all around her, and what she did to hide her monthly cycle, simply beggars belief.

The Battle of Schellenberg in Bavaria, took place on 2 July 1704, between the Grand Alliance of England, the Dutch Republic and Austria, against the smaller Army of King Louis XIV's forces. During the fighting, Christian was wounded when she was struck by a musket ball in the thigh. Despite her wound she continued to fight and was with the Duke of Marlborough's forces at the Battle of Blenheim, which took place the following month on 13 August, and resulted in a decisive victory for the Grand Alliance.

After the battle she was detailed to look after some of the French prisoners. Remarkably, it was whilst engaged in this duty, and after nearly 13 years of searching, that she saw her husband, Richard, who was serving with the 1st Regiment of Foot. Unfortunately for him he was in the process of chatting to a woman in circumstances other than might suggest that they were engaged in a conversation on the subject of military tactics. Despite Christian's anger at her husband's apparent philandering, they agreed not to reveal her secret of being a woman, and to cover the fact that they were often seen in each other's company, they pretended to be brothers, which nobody questioned.

The Battle of Ramillies in present day Belgium village of Walloon Brabant, took place on 23 May 1706. During the fighting Christian sustained a fractured skull. Because of this injury, and after nine years of keeping up her pretence of being a man, her lie was finally uncovered. Whilst treating her injuries the regimental surgeon discovered that Christopher Welsh was actually a woman. Such a matter would always be hard to keep a secret and it wasn't long before it came to the attention of the Scots Greys' commanding officer, Lord Hay. Both Christian and her husband Richard were brought before him to explain their story. Despite her military career being at an end, Lord Hay decided that her pay as a soldier should be continued whilst she was recovering from her injuries and receiving medical attention from the Army.

Once recovered she was formally discharged from the Scots Greys but was allowed to be carried on the strength of the 1st Regiment of Foot, as she was the wife of one of its soldiers. She carried out the useful service of being a sutleress, which was a civilian merchant who travelled with the Army and sold provisions to soldiers who were operating in the field.

Despite being reunited with his wife, in Marian Broderick's 2004 book, *Wild Irish Women*, it is clear that Richard did not change his ways where women were concerned. She describes how on finding out that one of her husband's mistresses was still travelling with the regiment, Christian viciously attacked the woman, cutting off her nose.

On 11 September 1709, the Battle of Malplaquet in France took place, and although deemed to be a victory for the forces of the Grand Alliance, it was a pyrrhic one due to the large number of casualties they sustained. It was during the fighting that Richard, Christian's husband was killed.

On hearing of his death she scoured the battlefield to find his body so that she could bury him.

Soon after Richard's death, Christian became involved in a relationship with Captain Ross, an officer in her old regiment, the Scots Greys, but despite this, and within just three months of her husband's death, she married another man, who was also serving with the Scots Greys, Dragoon Hugh Jones. Sadly, he was killed only a matter of months later at the siege of the Fort at Saint-Venant, in the Pas de Calais region of France.

As the War of the Spanish Succession began to wind down, Christian returned home, by which time her story was well-known by all classes of British society. She was even presented at the court of Queen Anne, who granted her a bounty of £50 and a shilling a day for the rest of her life.

In 1713 she returned to Ireland, where she opened a pub with her third husband who also had the surname of Davies. In her later years she was admitted to the Royal Hospital at Chelsea as one of its in-pensioners, quite possibly its first ever women. She died there on 7 July 1739 at the age of 72, and was buried in the hospital's small cemetery, with full military honours.

Hannah Snell was born on 23 April 1723 in Worcester. In 1740 and at just 17 years of age she made her way to London to make her fortune, or

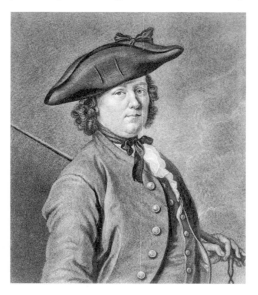

so it seemed. Four years later she was a wife, having married James Summes on 18 January 1744. When Hannah found herself pregnant with her husband's child early in the relationship, James Summes' response wasn't one of joy and celebration, and he certainly didn't act like a gentleman. Instead he walked out on Hannah.

The child, a daughter named Susannah, was born in 1746 in London, but sadly died when she was just one year old. How or of what she died from, history

Figure 50: Hannah Snell.

has not recorded, but a variety of diseases were rife in London at the time. Hannah must have been a determined individual, as she certainly didn't sit round feeling sorry for herself, instead she borrowed a man's suit from her brother-in-law, James Gray, and took his name. Then she went looking for her errant husband, whom it is said she discovered had been executed for murder.

I checked the list of executions for 1746 and 1747, on the website www. britishexecutions.co.uk, and there was no trace of the name James Summes. Either he wasn't executed for murder as is suggested on the Wikipedia entry for Hannah Snell, or he was hanged for murder, but under another name. Throughout Britain in 1745 a total of 31 men and women were hanged for their crimes. In 1746 a total of 116 men and women were hanged and in 1747 that number had fallen to just 46.

Soon after the death of her daughter, Hannah Snell moved to Portsmouth and, having kept up her pretence of being a man, managed to fool the authorities and enlist as a marine. On 23 October 1747, dressed in her marine's uniform, she boarded HMS *Swallow*, which was a 14-gun *Merlin* class sloop of wooden construction. She sailed for Lisbon, in Portugal, where they arrived on 1 November 1747, before continuing on to India, with her secret still intact.

As is the case when writing about historical events that occurred more than 250 years ago, establishing the facts isn't an exact science. Part of Hannah Snell's story is that in August 1748 she was sent on an expedition to capture the French colony of Pondicherry off the Carnatic coast of India. But the Battle of Pondicherry, didn't take place until 10 September 1759, some ten years later.

However, she did take part in the Battle of Devakottai in the state of Tamil Nadu, on the east coast of India, in June 1749 where she was wounded multiple times in the legs. One of the bullets struck her in the groin, but so as not to give away her secret, rather than be seen by the Army surgeon, she went to a local Indian woman to get her to remove the musket ball.

On her return to England in 1750 she decided to reveal to her shipmates that she was a woman, a secret she had hidden for over two years. She chose her moment well, on 2 June 1750 she was in a public house in London along with her colleagues from the Royal Marines when she broke the news.

They were supportive of her situation and encouraged her to seek a pension from the Duke of Cumberland, who was head of the English Army, although it should be pointed out that the Royal Marines are actually part of the Royal Navy and not the British Army. Hannah took her colleagues' advice, and two weeks later she approached the Duke of Cumberland whilst he was inspecting troops in St James's Park, London on 16 June 1750. Having presented the duke with a petition in relation to her request for an Army pension, she took a few minutes to avail him of her numerous military exploits.

She sold her story to Robert Walker, a London publisher, who printed her tales in a publication entitled, *The Female Soldier*.

Five months later Hannah Snell was informed by the Royal Hospital Chelsea of their acceptance of her military service and she was granted an Army pension for the rest of her life, which in her case was for a further forty years. During this time she married twice, first in 1759 to Richard Eyles, with whom she had two children, and in 1772 she married Richard Hapgood, both men living in Berkshire.

Unfortunately, over time her mental health deteriorated and in 1791 she was admitted to the Bedlam Lunatic Asylum, also known as the Bethlem Royal Hospital, at Bromley, in South London which is still open today. It first opened its doors as a Priory in 1247 and then became a hospital in 1330.

Hannah Snell is listed as one of the hospital's most notable patients, along with four others who attempted to assassinate King George III, one who set fire to York Minster and another who attempted to murder Queen Victoria and Prince Albert.

Chapter 13

Hansard Discussions

Over the years the Royal Hospital Chelsea has been the focus of many discussions by Members of Parliament in the House of Commons. Such discussions are recorded in Hansard, which keeps the official records of debates held in Parliament. I have included the content of some of these discussions on the following pages.

On **5 April 1807** Colonel Lockwood the MP for Epping in Essex, asked the following question in the House of Commons, of the Under Secretary of State for War: 'I beg to ask the Under of Secretary of State for War the number of men discharged, at their own request, from Chelsea Royal Hospital in each year from 1790 to the present time.'

Mr William Broderick, the Under Secretary of State for War and the Member of Parliament for Whitchurch in Hampshire, replied that in the seven years ending 1796 the numbers of pensioners discharged from Chelsea Hospital at their own request had been, 9, 17, 13, 13, 12, 24,18, a total of 106. He added that there were at the time a total of 547 in-pensioner's resident at the hospital.

Colonel Lockwood, still referring to the Royal Hospital but changing direction slightly, then fired a question in a most eloquent manner, at the Financial Secretary to the War office, in which he wanted to know how many contractors were employed to provide meat for the pensioners at the Royal Hospital Chelsea; and if the contract specifically stipulated that the meat had to be of English origin.

Mr J. Powell-Williams, explained that one contractor supplied the Royal Hospital Chelsea, but that the Infirmary contract was sometimes given to a separate firm, who to his knowledge only supplied best quality English meat.

Colonel Lockwood asked Mr Powell-Williams if he was aware that there were in fact two contractors involved in the supply of meat to the hospital. One being the person with whom the contract had been agreed with by the

Government, and the other being a sub-contractor who actually supplied the meat.

Mr Powell-Williams stated that he hadn't been aware of a sub-contractor being involved in the supply of meat to the hospital. As far as he had been aware there had only been the individual who had been contracted to do so by the Government.

Colonel Lockwood pushed the point, asking if Mr Powell-Williams would enquire into the matter, who replied that he would be more than happy to do so if the colonel provided him with the particulars of the case.

Captain Donelan, the MP for Cork East, asked who was responsible for seeing that the meat that was provided was of a sufficient standard, to which Mr Powell-Williams replied, that responsibility lay with the senior officer at the hospital, which quite possibly meant the Commissioners.

On **27 March 1873**, the MP for Devon and Eastern, Sir Lawrence Palk, asked the Secretary of State for War, Mr Edward Cardwell, if he would state to the House, why no steps had been taken, since the Royal Commission of 1870, to ascertain the wishes of the Chelsea Pensioners, to remain or leave. He further asked if it was true that a pensioner by the name of Kirk, who lived in the hospital's left wing, had received a punishment of seven day's confinement, for committing 'the crime' of sharing his regulation loaf of bread with his 72-year-old wife. He also asked whether there was a sergeant who was a resident of the hospital, who had been removed from Millbank for being too harsh with some of the persons under his charge.

Mr Cardwell provided a detailed reply. He informed Sir Lawrence that the inquiry of 1870 was not conducted by a Royal Commission, but by a departmental committee. It did not recommend, as Sir Lawrence appeared to believe, that any steps should be taken to ascertain the wishes of the pensioners to remain or leave. No married, or in-pensioner for that matter, is required to remain in the institution. Resumption of life as an out-pensioner at any time, is freely allowed. The pensioners are fully aware of this and a few of their number avail themselves of this right every year.

Mr Cardwell informed Sir Lawrence that no in-pensioner by the name of Kirk had been punished for sharing his regulation loaf of bread with his wife. But that a pensioner of that same name was confined to the hospital for a period of seven days for attempting to take away fuel which belonged to the hospital and to take his food outside at a forbidden hour. Mr Kirk had, on his admission to the hospital, stated that he had no relative who was dependent on him. Despite this untruth, Mr Kirk was allowed a pass to take food to his wife at the proper hour.

Mr Cardwell also confirmed that no sergeant or other person who was removed from Millbank for being too severe with his pensioners, was subsequently employed at the Royal Hospital Chelsea. There had been a sergeant of Police who was formerly employed at Millbank, but he voluntarily resigned his position, and left with a good character and his name and reputation intact.

On **13 September 1887** there was a discussion in Parliament about the Royal Hospital Chelsea and who was employed to work there.

Sir Henry Tyler, the Conservative Member of Parliament for Great Yarmouth between 1885 and 1892, had previously served as an officer in the Royal Engineers for some 24 years and the Inspector Officer of Railways, his work taking him all over the world. He asked a question of Mr Stanhope, the Secretary of State for War, whether it was the case in Naval Hospitals that Army Pensioners are employed as male nurses, and whether there is any objection to the employment at the Royal Hospital Chelsea, of pensioners from the Royal Marines or the Royal Navy, if they were qualified or suited for a particular job of work. He also asked, whether, as would appear to be the case, from a letter dated 6 September 1887, and sent by the Lieutenant Governor of the Royal Hospital Chelsea, where he states, 'it is absolutely the rule that Naval or Royal Marine pensioners are not eligible for employment in the Royal Hospital Chelsea.'

In response Mr Stanhope said that Chelsea Hospital, differs altogether in character from the Naval Hospitals. The latter are merely for the treatment of the sick; whereas Chelsea is a home for aged soldiers. The rule is that employment at the hospital shall be limited to Army Pensioners, whose numbers are very large. He did not believe that the rules could be altered without great inconvenience.

On **24 February 1896** a question was asked of the Under Secretary of State for War, by the MP for Chelsea, Mr Charles Whitmore. He wanted to know if the Commissioners of the Royal Hospital Chelsea, had made arrangements for compensation to be afforded to the in-pensioners at the hospital, in consequence of the withdrawal in June 1895, of the privilege, which they had enjoyed for more than 200 years, of being allowed to sell their old uniforms once they needed replacing.

Mr Broderick replied that arrangements had been made to give an annual grant of 7s to each of the hospital's in-pensioners, who were affected by the new change which forbade them from selling off their old clothing. In essence this meant that all future in-pensioners, and those who became residents of the hospital, after 22 June 1895, would not be entitled to the same grant as they had never been in the position of being able to sell their old uniforms.

On **22 March 1911** there was a very brief exchange in Parliament between Mr William Crooks, the MP for Woolwich, and the Home Secretary, Mr Winston Churchill.

Mr Crooks asked the Home Secretary whether he would take steps to secure the grant of a free pardon for ex-sergeant Price, who had recently been released from prison, and on whose behalf a petition had been presented to the House of Commons, signed by more than 70,000 people. This would enable Price to resume his Army pension, monies which he was in dire need of.

Mr Churchill replied that he could not find sufficient grounds that would warrant the granting of a free pardon in this matter. It would not affect the question of the restoration of his pension, which was a matter in the discretion of the Commissioners of the Royal Hospital Chelsea.

Despite Mr Churchill's comments in the House of Commons that day, it would appear that he had a change of heart, because by 20 May 1911, just two months later, Price was granted a pardon by the king.

It was reported that the king, had, on the advice of the Home Secretary, Mr Winston Churchill, agreed to grant a free pardon to John Price, formerly a sergeant with the 3rd (Volunteer) Battalion, Queen's Own (Royal West Kent Regiment) who in 1902 was convicted of the murder of his wife by shooting her in the canteen of the Drill Hall, Beresford Street, Woolwich, on Saturday, 21 September 1901. Sergeant John Price was the canteen sergeant and officer's steward at the Drill Hall. On the day before the murder, Price and his wife, Barbara, had argued in the canteen about their son. On the day of the murder the argument had continued, with the couple verbally going at each other on about three occasions before Price shot Barbara with a single shot from his army rifle. His trial took place at the Central Criminal Courts of the Old Bailey. On its conclusion on Saturday, 26 October 1901, Price was found guilty of murder.

His conviction should have seen him executed, but his sentence of death was commuted to penal servitude for life by the Judge, Mr Justice Bigham. Price was eventually released on licence in October 1910.

Price's pardon meant that his name was restored to the Army Pension list. The act of murdering his wife was done so under extreme provocation by her and had been described as being 'extenuating circumstances'.

In June 1902, Lord Charles Beresford MP presented a petition of some 10,000 names to the Home Secretary, asking him to reconsider the case of Sergeant John Price. In response the Home Secretary wrote to Price's solicitor, Mr Llewellyn Davies, to inform him that he had fully considered the case and regretted that he was unable to consider any remission of his client's sentence.

On his eventual release from prison, Price returned to living at his old home in Woolwich where he was still exceedingly popular, and a man for whom there was a great deal of sympathy, but by May 1911 he had sailed to Canada on the Allan liner *Vittorian*, to start a new life. With the help of Norman Gzowski, the nephew of the late General Sandham, Price had been appointed the manager of a 400-acre farm near Toronto. He had been born and raised on a farm in England and saw his move to Canada as a fresh start. Others had supported him during his time of incarceration, including the Conservative MP, Major William Augustus Adams who, for a brief period of time between January and December 1910, represented Woolwich in the House of Commons, and time after time brought Price's circumstances to the attention of his fellow MPs.

Why Winston Churchill changed his mind on the matter is not known, and whether the Commissioners of the Royal Hospital Chelsea had used their discretion to restore Price's pension before or after the king had granted him a pardon, is something that I have not been able to establish.

On **23 October 1912** the MP for St Augustine's, Mr Ronald McNeil, asked a question of the Secretary of State for War in relation to military pensions, concerning a specific individual.

Frederick Ribbens, a retired sergeant of the York and Lancaster Regiment, had served in the British Army for more than thirteen years and if he had served for just a further eight months he would have been entitled to a pension for life. But in June 1909 he was medically discharged because he contracted rheumatic fever whilst serving in India and his feet became so weak that he was deemed to be medically unfit for further military service.

His conduct and character were marked as being exemplary, but despite this he was certainly done no favours. Instead of a pension for life, he ended up with a temporary one of 10d per day for thirty-nine months. He originally enlisted in the Army as a band boy at such an age as prevented him from learning a trade. Sergeant Ribbens was a married man with children.

Because of Sergeant Ribbens' situation, Mr McNeil, reminded the Secretary of State for War, that Ribbens was in a difficult predicament of not being able to work because of an ailment he acquired during his service in the British Army whilst stationed in India. Mr McNeil added that in the circumstances he hoped the Secretary of State for War would arrange for Ribbens to be awarded a full pension.

The reply which Mr McNeil received was not the one that he or ex-sergeant Ribbens were hoping for. Mr Harold Baker, the Secretary of State for War, stated, that the disability for which Ribbens was discharged from the Army, could not be attributed to the effects of climate or military service, which meant that Commissioners of the Royal Hospital Chelsea, were therefore not in a position to increase his pension, as he had already been awarded the maximum pension that he was entitled to. It was a decision that appeared to be somewhat harsh back in 1912, an opinion which the passage of time hasn't done much to alter.

On **17 July 1916** Mr Crean, the MP for Cork South East, asked the Secretary of State for War to look into the case of Gunner 2898, Michael Hurley, who had served with the Royal Garrison Artillery, and who lived at Rock Street, Kinsale, County Cork. Gunner Hurley lost a leg from the thigh down during fighting at Hill 60, France, which took place between 17 to 22 April 1915 and

1 to 7 May 1915. So fierce was the fighting for Hill 60, that three British officers and two soldiers were awarded the Victoria Cross for their actions.

Gunner Hurley had been awarded a small pension of 10s 6d. Mr Crean was asking that consideration be given for it to be raised, because not only had he been crippled by his wartime service, but he had an elderly mother and an invalid brother who were both dependent on him. Mr Crean reminded the Secretary of State for War that other wounded soldiers who had been similarly circumstanced, were in receipt of pensions of 14s and more.

Mr Forster replied that Gunner Hurley's pension had been increased from 10s 6d to 12s 6d per week and reminded Mr Crean that the Commissioners of the Royal Hospital Chelsea had no power to increase a soldier's pension in relation to dependants, unless they were children.

Mr Crean countered by asking the Secretary of State for War if he believed that the mentioned increase in Gunner Hurley's pension would be sufficient for him, his mother and brother.

Mr Forster stated that if Gunner Hurley, or anybody acting on his behalf, wrote to the Secretary of the Royal Hospital Chelsea, full consideration would be given to his case.

Mr Butcher, the MP for York, enquired of Mr Forster whether the Statutory Committee could give some increase to the man's pension. Mr Forster replied that they could if such a request was made to them and that they felt such an increase was merited.

On **19 July 1916** in the House of Commons, a question was asked by Mr Ellis Hume-Williams, MP for Bassetlaw, of the Secretary of State for War, Mr Henry Forster, in relation to the on-going medical treatment for discharged wounded soldiers, who had served their king and country.

The question was whether soldiers who had been discharged from the Army, and awarded a pension on account of the wounds they received whilst on active service, were left to pay out of their own pocket for any subsequent medical treatment that their wounds might require; and if that were the case, would provision be made for free treatment for those individuals who suffered as a direct result of wounds received during the war?

Mr Forster replied that soldiers discharged from the Army on account of wounds can, on application to the secretary of the Royal Hospital Chelsea, obtain treatment in a military hospital provided there is a reasonable probability that their disability will be cured or materially improved. While a patient at the hospital the man's pension is raised to the full amount which is allowed for total disablement and any allowance for children who were born before the man was discharged, to which they might be entitled. A stoppage of one shilling per day is made to cover the cost of them being a patient at the hospital.

Mr Hume-Williams asked if the same arrangements might not be made available to men who lived in country districts, and who were possibly less mobile, and not readily able to get to the Royal Hospital Chelsea.

Mr Forster replied that such a suggestion was agreeable and that the same arrangement would apply with accommodation being found for these men in the most convenient and closest military hospital. Any such application had to, in the first instance, be made in writing to the Secretary of the Royal Hospital Chelsea.

Sir Clement Kinloch-Cooke, who was at the time the MP for Devonport, became involved in the discussion when he asked the question of Mr Forster, as to whether a wife and child were still in receipt of an Army pension whilst their husband/father was in hospital being treated. Mr Forster explained that in such circumstances, the dependent's pension is raised to the maximum amount allowed under the pension rules.

Mr Forster was at pains to explain that the circumstances he was talking about, only related to men who had already been discharged from the Army and then had a subsequent medical issue, which was connected to the wounds which they had originally received. He added that no man wounded in action or otherwise in need of hospital treatment whilst in military service, would be discharged from the Army until after the treatment of their initial wounds was complete.

On **18 November 1919** the MP for Chelsea, Lieutenant-Colonel Sir Samuel Hoare, asked the Secretary of State for War, whether a decision had been made in relation to the hardship experienced by in-pensioners at the Royal Hospital Chelsea, by the loss of their out-pension when they become resident at the hospital?

Mr Henry Forster confirmed that no in-pensioner at the Royal Hospital Chelsea would be affected by the new scale of Army pensions, since its application is confined to those who have actually given military service during the war, and in any case, under the terms of the Soldiers' Pensions Act 1928, veterans who were admitted to the hospital as in-pensioners did so knowing that by the terms of their admittance, their Army pensions were abrogated, meaning the point that Sir Samuel had made, was not relevant.

Sir Samuel, perhaps caught off guard by Mr Forster's response, pushed the matter asking had Mr Forster, some three months earlier, fielded the same question by promising an enquiry would be held into the matter. Mr Forster confirmed such an enquiry was underway, which would hopefully be completed in a few week's time.

On **8 July 1924** the MP for Ashton-under-Lyne, Colonel Sir Walter de Frece, asked a question of the Secretary of State for War, Mr Stephen Walsh, if he would specify the exact type of pension claims which were dealt with by the Royal Hospital Chelsea authorities.

Mr Stephen Walsh explained that the Commissioners of the Royal Hospital dealt with all awards to warrant officers, non-commissioned officers and men of the Army, of pensions earned by service, including long-service pensions, campaign pensions and pensions awarded for gallant conduct. They also dealt with awards of pensions to those ranks in respect of disablement due to wound, injury or disease, that were attributable to military service in peace and in any war subsequent to the Great War. But where the disablement was incurred during the Great War, or in former wars, the pension was dealt with by the Ministry of Pensions. Any subsequent claims for an increase or commutation of any of the awards they were responsible for, were also dealt with by the Commissioners of the Royal Hospital Chelsea.

Another sad case involving the Royal Hospital Chelsea, an ex-soldier and an issue about the man's hope that he would be looked after having served his country was raised on **6 March 1928**.

Mr L'Estrange Malone posed the question concerning an ex-soldier and his pension. The man in question was Mr George Frederick Mackenzie, who had previously served as Private 28884 with the Northampton Territorial Force. When he had signed up he was passed A1 fit in relation to his health. The same outcome was recorded in May 1924 when he enlisted in the

Regular Army. Some time after this date he was admitted to hospital for treatment but was discharged after receiving treatment for five days. Shortly after this he was on a period of leave when he was taken ill and admitted to Northampton Hospital and was found to be suffering from consumption. He was invalided out of the Army in June 1927.

Despite having served for three years by the time he was discharged, George Mackenzie was refused a pension although he was unable to work because of his consumption. This was not an illness which ran in the family and Mr Mackenzie's own father was himself a retired soldier. Mr Malone wanted to know if there was any right of appeal to the Commissioners of the Royal Hospital Chelsea, against their decision that his illness was a non-attributable disability.

Mr Duff Cooper, the Financial Secretary to the War Office, provided the following response. He confirmed that Mr Mackenzie's case was referred by the Commissioners of the Royal Hospital Chelsea, to the Director General of Army Medical Services, who was the ultimate medical authority on such matters. Having considered all the available information the Director General confirmed the decision which had previously been made by the Commissioners and determined that Mr Mackenzie's disability was not attributable to military service. There was no right of appeal to this decision.

On **21 May 1931** a very brief exchange took place in Parliament concerning the Royal Hospital Chelsea. Sir Samuel Hoare, the Secretary of State for India, asked whether there was a proposal in the offing to sell off or let the Royal Hospital Chelsea's burial ground. Mr Thomas Shaw, the Secretary of State for War, and the MP for Preston, replied that the burial ground at the Royal Hospital Chelsea, belonged to the Commissioners of the Hospital, and that there were no proposals under consideration to either sell or let the burial grounds.

On **5 November 1936** one of the topics being discussed in Parliament concerned campaign pensions. Mr Thomas Williams, the MP for Don Valley, asked the Secretary of State for War, whether he was aware of the difficulties some retired soldiers were experiencing when they tried to apply for a special campaign pension on reaching the national retirement age of 65. Many of them had been obliged to apply for public assistance before their pension was awarded, which threw up another problem, that as long as they were receiving public assistance, their eagerly anticipated pension was withheld.

Mr Williams asked the Secretary of State if he would arrange to have this extremely unhelpful anomaly, removed. A solution to the problem he could see as workable, would be to award such special pensions two months before the men reached the age of 65.

Mr Cooper, the Secretary of State for War stated that it was already the practice of the Commissioners of the Royal Hospital Chelsea to consider applications for Special Campaign pensions which are submitted shortly before the date on which the claimant attains the required age.

On **29 April 1941** Sir John Smedley Crooke, the Conservative MP for Birmingham Deritend, asked the Secretary of State for War, Captain David Margesson, whether or not any provision had been made for the free supply, repair and renewals of artificial limbs in the cases of soldiers who lost a limb or limbs whilst serving in the British Army, and in whose cases there is no entitlement to pension on grounds that disability is not directly attributable to military service.

Captain David Margesson, who besides being the Secretary of State for War, was also the MP for Rugby, replied that in such cases an artificial limb is supplied by the Royal Hospital Chelsea, through the Ministry of Pensions, and repairs and renewals may be allowed at the discretion of the Commissioners of the Royal Hospital.

On **8 February 1944** a discussion took place in Parliament on the subject of Boer War Pensioners. Sir Geoffrey Shakespeare, the MP for Norwich, asked the Secretary of State for War, Sir James Grigg, a two–part question, the first part of which was, what were the number of pensions granted and administered by the Royal Hospital Chelsea in respect of disabilities attributable to the Boer War; and what was the annual sum of money involved? Secondly, whether he would secure for the Boer War pensioners, whose pensions are administered by the Royal Hospital Chelsea, the benefits secured by Parliament and operated through the Ministry of Pensions for pensioners of the Great War 1914–1918 and of the Second World War.

Sir James Grigg replied that the bulk of the Boer War disability pensions were administered by the Right Hon. Minister of Pensions. The few that were administered by the Royal Hospital Chelsea, were in respect of belated claims with which I understand my right hon. friend is unable to deal. The awards made by the Royal Hospital are made under the Boer War regulations which in most cases has seen an increase of 70 per cent over Boer War rates. Sir James finished by saying that he was considering whether the basis of the award could be revised.

Sir Geoffrey Shakespeare asked whether Sir James would take into account the fact that the Boer War pensioner has his disability pension reduced when he undertakes light work.

Sir James Grigg promised that he would look in to the disparity of the pension amounts and was quite willing to take into account any factors that were brought to his notice in relation to the matter.

Major General Sir Alfred Knox, the conservative MP for Wycombe, asked Sir James Grigg if it were not possible for him to provide the House with a figure of the total amount spent in a year on the pensions in question, and, in view of that amount, were it not possible to increase the pensions further.

Sir James Grigg, re-iterated his position and already stated commitment to look into the whole basis of the awards in question. Other than that, there was no more he could say on the matter.

On **27 January 1947** there was a brief discussion concerning the purchase of some beds for the Royal Hospital Chelsea.

Colonel George Wigg posed a question to the Minister of Works, Mr George Tomlinson, concerning the purchase of beds. He wanted to know why, when there was a shortage of beds, had the hospital invited tenders for some 300 special beds for use in the Royal Hospital Chelsea, when there was clearly a large number of surplus beds available in the aftermath of the war.

Mr Tomlinson replied, informing Colonel Wigg that the standard wartime bed did not fit into the individual ward cubicles where the in-pensioners slept. In particular, they were deemed to be insufficiently wide enough for the men's needs.

On hearing Mr Tomlinson's detailed reply, Colonel Wigg did not take the matter any further, one supposes because he was suitably satisfied with the answer.

On **17 February 1953** Mr Edward Short, the MP for Newcastle-upon-Tyne Central asked the Secretary of State for War if he would take steps to see that crosses properly inscribed are provided for all Chelsea Pensioners buried in Brookwood Cemetery.

Mr James Hutchison, the Under Secretary for War and the MP for Glasgow Scotstoun, replied that the pensioners and staff of the Royal Hospital Chelsea are buried in a special plot and are commemorated by a central memorial.

Mr Short asked whether it was not a shocking disgrace that these fine old pensioners should have their graves marked only by a peg in the ground with a number attached to it, especially as there are a short distance away neat, well-kept graves of Poles and Czechs tended by the Imperial War Graves Commission? Mr Short asked Mr Hutchison if he would have the pensioners' graves transferred so that they were tended by the Imperial War Graves Commission, allowing them to be cared for in a similar manner.

Mr Hutchison: '*I would point out that there is a fine central memorial to all the Chelsea Pensioners. There are opportunities for Pensioners to make comments upon this, but they have never done so, nor have their relations. If relations wish to provide for a burial outside the cemetery, it is open to them to do so, and they get financial aid. Furthermore, if a relative wanted to erect a cross of this kind, he would be allowed to do so in consultation with the authorities.*'

Mr Short: '*Does not the Minister realise that these old Chelsea Pensioners are buried in a rough, uneven bit of ground in Brookwood Cemetery and that each grave is marked only by a peg with a number on it? Does he not regard that as shocking?*'

Sir Fitzroy Maclean, the MP for Lancaster, who in 1954 would go on to become the Financial Secretary to the War Office, asked Mr Hutchison about the costs involved in such a proposal.

Mr Hutchison: '*About £10 to £12 each. The funds of the Chelsea Hospital are not excessive, and we believe it is better to expend them on the living.*'

Mr George Wigg, the MP for Dudley in the West Midlands, and who in 1967 would become Lord Wigg, entered the affray. '*Does the hon. Gentleman realise that the Government are making money of the Chelsea Pensioners? Before a man becomes an inmate of the Royal Chelsea Hospital he has to surrender his pension. Would it not be only decent to give back some of that money in order to erect at least a headstone?*'

Mr Hutchison: *'I shall have a look in to that aspect.'*
Mr Short: *'It may be a small thing, but I regard it as a minor national disgrace. I beg to give notice that I will raise the matter on the Adjournment.'*

On **8 June 1962** a very interesting debate took place concerning the Royal Hospital Chelsea. The question was brought to the House by the MP for Chelsea, Captain John Litchfield. The purpose of the debate was to discuss damage caused to the hospital's buildings during the Second World War. Captain Litchfield outlined that in February 1918, during the First World War, the hospital's north-east wing was destroyed in a daytime air raid by German Zeppelins. The extensive damage caused in this raid was eventually repaired three years later in 1921.

He then drew a comparison with the damage once again caused to the north-east wing in 1944, when it was struck by a German V2 rocket, and pointed out that eighteen years later, the damaged edifice had still not been repaired to its former glory.

Captain Litchfield then set out what he hoped would be his persuasive argument for the expedient repair of this iconic building. He started off by pointing out how it must have looked to visitors to London seeing such a noble and historic building in the nation's capital, still looking like a derelict bomb site, whilst nearby new office blocks and hotels were being erected at will.

He then pointed out that there were 410 in-pensioners who were residents of the Royal Hospital, and a waiting list of about 100 who were waiting to join them. This led him nicely into explaining the urgent nature, as he saw it, of rebuilding the north-east wing, so that much needed accommodation could be provided for some of the more infirm and elderly in-pensioners, those who perhaps did not need full hospital treatment, but who needed greater care and attention than was available at the time in the day to day life of the Royal Hospital. With the north-east wing rebuilt, there would be sufficient room to include two more wards which would mean enough accommodation for some 65 more in-pensioners

He spoke out of the social aspects which extended far beyond the walls of the Royal Hospital, as many of the aforementioned pensioners would have at the time been living in circumstances of personal hardship and distress in various parts of the country, not just to themselves but those with whom they were living.

Captain Litchfield reminded his fellow MPs that they often directed their attention and sympathies towards the problems which faced society's old and infirm, and discussed the issues of distress and loneliness that they faced if not properly cared for, and the issues which arose for those called upon or expected to look after them through such difficult times.

He then addressed the issue of the cost of such a build, pointing out that currently a conservative estimate would be somewhere in the region of £83,000. If it had been carried out say ten years earlier that figure may well have been closer to £50,000, and if it was left for a few more years, then the figure could easily rise to around the £100,000. The feeling from Government was that they did not feel such expenditure on making good the damage to the north-east wing of the Royal Hospital Chelsea, could be justified when balanced against the state of the national economy at the time.

Captain Litchfield, with all the sharpness and attention to detail normally attributed to a skilled lawyer, made reference to the grants available under the Historic Buildings and Ancient Monuments Act 1953, drawing comparisons with the cost of the needed repairs to the Royal Hospital, when compared as a percentage of the expenditure voted for the upkeep of ancient monuments for the financial year 1962–63, which was in the region of some £900,000, yet not one penny of that could be spared for repairs to the north-east wing of the Royal Hospital.

But he wasn't stopping there. Captain Litchfield then made mention of the new Army barracks being built just across the road from the Royal Hospital at a cost of more than £2 million. At least that was for a building of purpose, but his argument was put into perspective when he made mention of the £2 million Supplementary Estimate for Government stationery and printing, taking into account that this was on top of the £6 million already agreed for the same items.

He guessed that one of the arguments that would be put up as a reason for not meeting the costs of undertaking the rebuilding of the Royal Hospital, would be priorities, which allowed him to say that was his very point. By failing to acknowledge the urgency of these repairs when compared to the expenditure he had mentioned, the Government had its priorities in the wrong order.

Captain Litchfield then took a look at how successive Governments had dealt with the issue, despite Governors of the Royal Hospital having pushed for the work to be completed. In 1952 the then Minister of Works visited the hospital and actually expressed his concern at the absence of the wing, and despite agreeing to 'tackle the problem', nothing happened. In 1954 the Hospital's Governor, General Sir Bernard Paget GCB MC, visited the Minister of Works, only for him to explain that they were targeting their available resources on the hospital's new Infirmary. On the one hand that was positive news, but it wasn't enough. In 1957 another Minister of Works visited the Royal Hospital, the outcome of which was, nothing.

In 1958 the hospital's new Governor, General Sir Cameron Nicholson GCB KBE DSO* MC* continued pushing for the work on the north-east wing to be completed. This time there was encouraging news. It was agreed that plans could go ahead and that work on the project was to begin in August 1961. Two months before this date the Royal Hospital was informed that £83,000 was to be included in the budget for the financial year 1962-63 so that the work could be completed in 1962. That news was made public on the day of the 1961 Founders' Day Parade by the Royal Hospital's Governor. At last there was a real ray of light at the end of the tunnel, or was there? No sooner had the first turf been dug in the rebuilding in September 1961, than a letter from the Ministry of Works was received by the Governor of the Royal Hospital, telling him that work on the planned rebuilding was to cease immediately so as to meet Treasury demands to curb expenditure, and by June 1962 that is where the situation stood.

After Captain Litchfield had finished his passionate and moving plea, it was the turn of Mr Richard Thompson, the Parliamentary Secretary to the Minister of Works to reply. He began in a complimentary and sympathetic manner, as Captain Litchfield had suggested he might, but that sympathy didn't last for long. Mr Thompson was quick to dismiss the comparison Captain Litchfield had made between the time it had taken to repair the north-east wing after the damage caused in the First World War, as to that caused during the Second World War. There was no comparison to be made he suggested, because the devastation caused by enemy air raids during the Second World War was far greater than anything that had happened during the First, but despite this, the Government had completed a tremendous amount of much needed work since the end of the last war, despite what Captain Litchfield saw as the Government not getting its priorities right.

Using boxing analogies, Mr Thompson stood his ground and fought his corner, and he certainly wasn't going down without a fight. He pointed out the monies which had been spent on the Royal Hospital, highlighting the cost of new and larger berths for the in-pensioners which had meant a reduction in their number, at a cost of £38,000. The steam-driven boiler which powered the hospital's heating system was renewed at a cost of a further £30,000. The kitchen was re-equipped and updated which cost £15,000, not to mention the £203,000 which it had cost to build the hospital's new Infirmary, one that he pointed out was one of the finest of its kind in the world. This, he said, was a fine example of just how well the Government had definitely got its priorities right. There was more that he could have mentioned, but he had no desire to go through what he called a long shopping list of items just to negate Captain Litchfield's accusations that Government wasn't doing enough when it came to the Royal Hospital. He added that the sum spent so far since the end of the war was some £385,000.

Mr Thompson was keen to point out that it wasn't just a case of throwing up some bricks and concrete to replicate what had gone before it, because not only was this an historic building, but it was one which had been built by Sir Christopher Wren and was one of his renowned masterpieces. He suggested that Captain Litchfield's figure for the cost of the work was a great deal higher than £83,000, and was more like £130,000, some £50,000 more.

He went on to say that he wished he could provide the categorical assurances that his 'honourable and gallant friend' so desperately wanted to hear would be included in the Budget for the period 1963-64, but he was not able to do so, and he understood that Captain Litchfield was not disposed to being fobbed off with sympathy, but that was the truth of the matter. He did add that much of the pre-contract work, which would have to be done in any case, was well under way, and to that extent things were moving forward.

Mr Thompson confirmed that the Government was anxious to reinstate the scheme that would see the rebuilding of the hospital's north-east wing, which would go ahead as soon as financial circumstances allowed it to. He stated that the decision to remove the allocated monies for the project from that year's budget was a decision that had been taken with the greatest of regret. He pointed out that, although he understood that his words were ultimately not what Captain Litchfield wanted to hear, and he could not give him any categorical assurances in relation to time scales for the completion of the hoped for works, he, Captain Litchfield, had achieved something for the cause he had at heart by having raised the matter so eloquently and passionately, and that what he had done 'today' would, he was sure, materially contribute to the speeding up of this project, which was what both of them ultimately wanted to happen.

Mr Hoy, the MP for Leith in Scotland, also spoke on the matter, which in the main was in support of Captain Litchfield.

Overall, Captain Litchfield and Mr Thompson engaged each other in an eloquent, respectful and dignified manner, not losing sight of what the real issue was. It wasn't party one-up-manship that was being played out, it was the heart and soul of the Royal Hospital Chelsea that was at stake, which neither man lost sight of, which was good to see.

On **23 May 1977** Mr David Price, the MP for Eastleigh, asked a question of, Mr Robert Brown, the Secretary of State for Defence, and also the MP for Newcastle-upon-Tyne, what costs were incurred by the Royal Hospital each year of the Royal Horticultural Society's Flower Show being held at the Royal Hospital, and how much the Society, the exhibitors and contractors contributed towards these costs.

Mr Brown replied that the Royal Horticultural Society pays a rental to the Commissioners for the use of the Royal Hospital's grounds to stage their annual show, and that the rehabilitation of the hospital grounds after the show has finished and the costs related to that, are the responsibility of the Society, meaning that the Royal Hospital did not incur any costs as a result of staging the flower show each year.

On **9 March 1982** the MP for the borough of Havering Upminster, Mr John Loveridge, asked the question of Mr Nott, the then Secretary of State for Defence. It is worth pointing out at this juncture that less than a month later, on 2 April, Argentinian forces invaded the Falkland Islands, so putting Britain on a war footing with Argentina. The question asked by Mr Loveridge was would the Secretary of State for Defence, make a statement on the funding of the Royal Hospital Chelsea.

Mr Nott replied as follows:

'*My department has reviewed, together with the Commissioners of the Royal Hospital Chelsea, the arrangements for funding and staffing the Hospital, which is a crown body administered by the commissioners under letters patent. We have decided that from 1 April 1982 the Royal Hospital will be funded by a block grant in aid instead of from a number of votes both within and outside the ambit of the Defence budget. This will enable expenditure on the Royal Hospital to be published in a more regular and identifiable way. The commissioners will have greater flexibility in staff management, including the freedom to fill vacancies either with staff employed directly by themselves or with staff on loan from the Ministry of Defence. The new arrangements are expected to improve the efficiency and economy of the Royal Hospital.*'

On **19 March 1990** a question was asked by Sir Michael McNair-Wilson, the MP for Newbury, of the Secretary of State for defence, Mr Archie Hamilton, about what qualified a person to be an occupant of the Royal Hospital Chelsea.

Mr Hamilton answered the question, informing Mr McNair-Wilson that those who are eligible for admittance are determined under the hospital's regulations which were issued under royal warrant. Former soldiers of the British Army, of good character, are eligible for admission to the Royal Hospital as an in-pensioner if they are in receipt of a service pension, or service invaliding pension which is paid for by the Ministry of Defence, and which was awarded in respect of service which included such period of service in the British Army, as the Hospital's Commissioners consider adequate.

It also includes a former soldier who has been awarded a disability pension by the Ministry of Defence or the Department of Social Security in respect of a disability which resulted from having served in the British Army. Those veterans who have been awarded a Victoria Cross or George Medal annuity which relates to acts of bravery whilst serving in the British Army, and who are not less than 65 years of age. Also included are those who are incapable of supplementing their pensions because of the loss of a limb, wounds or other accepted injuries, or disabilities which resulted from their service in the British Army.

There were a few other variables included in the admissions policy, most of which were at the discretion of the Hospital's Commissioners and were included in Mr Hamilton's full reply.

These examples are just a small number of the numerous discussions and debates which have taken place in the hallowed chambers of the House of Commons over the years, which relate in some way to the Royal Hospital Chelsea, highlighting in some ways, it could be argued, just how important an establishment it was, and still is to this day.

Chapter 14

Correspondence

Whilst researching this book we came across a few post cards and a letter connected to the Royal Hospital which are included here. The first was a letter written to Mr James Bostock of Bedford Row, Great Guildford Street, Southwark, formerly of the 95th Regiment of Foot. It is dated 26 May 1840 and reads as follows;

James Bostock,
In reply to your application of the 29th April, I have to acquaint you that it will be necessary for you to attend at this department for the purpose of undergoing an examination with the view of establishing your identity as the individual admitted on the Pension List.
Rich Newell, Secretary & Registrar.

A postcard of the Church of the Holy Sepulchre in Northampton, dated 30 September 1904, was sent to a young lady, who went by the name of Miss Bignell, with her address being the Governor's House, Royal Hospital, Chelsea, London SW. Bignell certainly wasn't the name of the governor at the time, who was Field Marshal Sir Henry Norman GCB GCMG CIE. The card reads as follows:

Dear 'L',
Have you had any news of 'S'. We have not had a line, and up to last Sunday, they had not heard at home. Hope you are well. Got back alright, do let us have a card, love to you and Mrs G. Have just wrote a card to Nell.
Clifford.

Another postcard was one sent from the Hotel Italie in Florence, Italy on 19 November 1907. The details of the person who sent it, aren't included, but it was sent to Mr Price, of Ward No.6, Royal Hospital Chelsea.

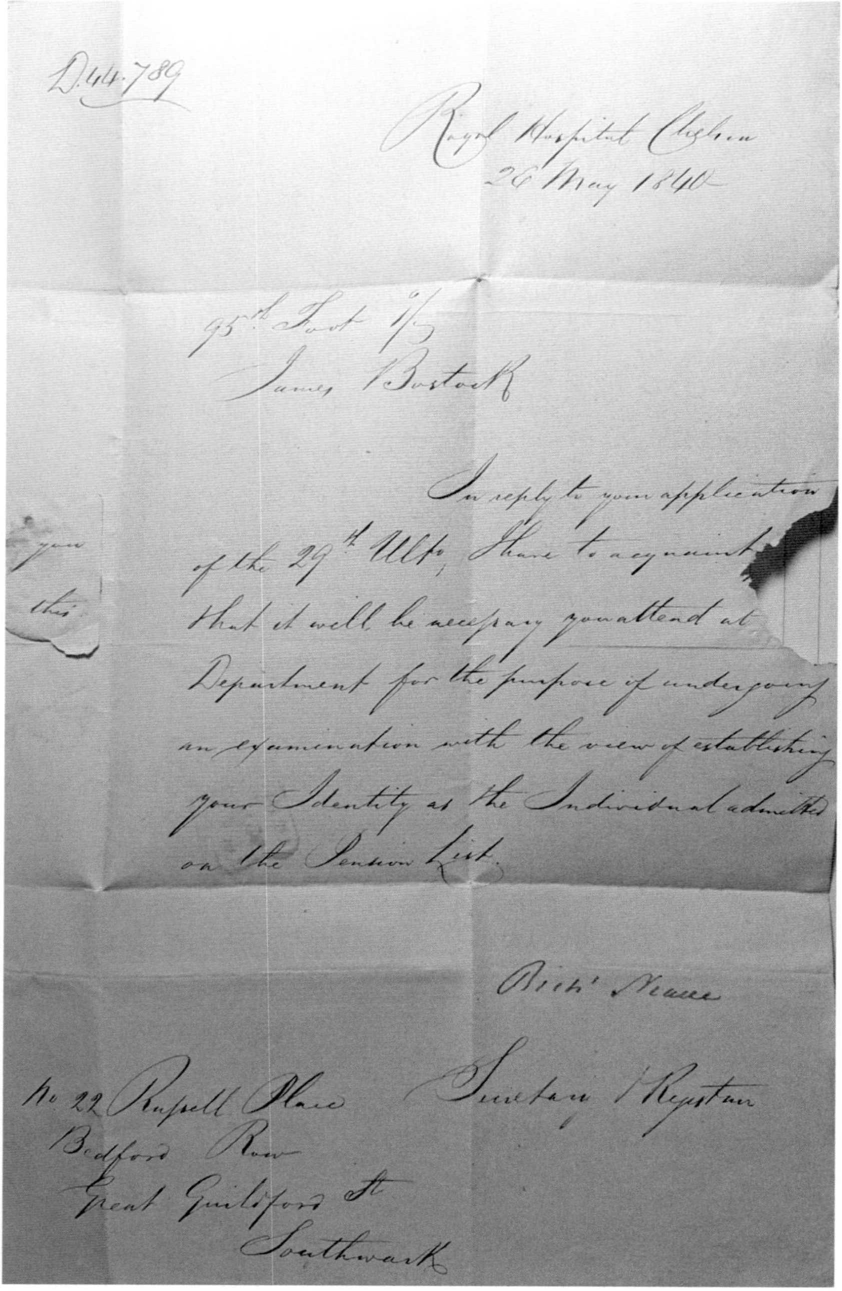

Figure 51: Letter to James Bostock.

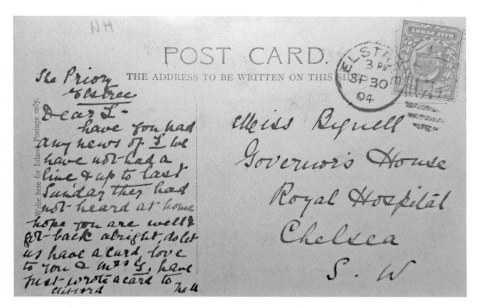

Figure 52: Rear of Post Card to Miss Bignell.

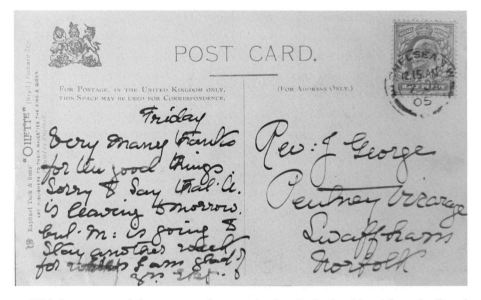

This is a post card that was sent by somebody who had paid a visit to the Royal hospital, we assume on 7 January 1905, as that is the day it was posted. It was sent to the Reverend J. George who lived at the Vicarage in Swaffham, Norfolk.

Conclusion

Hopefully this book has provided a flavour of the rich and varied history of the Royal Hospital Chelsea. What we have written only scratches the surface of the entire story, which goes to make up the history of the hospital's long and cherished existence. For us, it has been a really enjoyable experience writing this book, not only because of the stories and characters we have discovered from across the years, but because of the numerous visits we have made to the hospital and some of the people we have met who either work at, or are in-pensioners there.

It is incredible to think this is an institution which has been in continual existence since 1692, with 2017 seeing it celebrate its 325th anniversary. The fact that over the years, so many aged veterans from the British Army have had the opportunity to see out the twilight years of their lives in the comfortable, friendly and picturesque surroundings of the Royal Hospital Chelsea, is testament to the continued commitment and hard work of so many, in an establishment which has been governed and run by a Board of Commissioner since 1702. It has the added bonus of receiving an annual government grant which assists with its day-to-day running costs and is also an independent charity.

As retirement and nursing homes go, it not only possesses some of the most up-to-date equipment and accommodation in the world, but it also has some of the most highly dedicated and skilled members of staff that any organisation could possibly wish to have working for them.

Hopefully the hospital will go from strength to strength and continue to be part of the very fabric of everything that is good about this great nation. The hospital has remained an iconic establishment since it first opened its doors in 1692, and the scarlet tunics, tricorne hats, along with the in-pensioners who wear them, have ensured that its residents continue to possess the high status.

The Royal Hospital Chelsea has a very useful and helpful website (www.chelsea-pensioners.co.uk) which is full of information about its history, and the men and women who have lived and worked there. It also includes an on-line 'Book of Remembrance' which includes the names of 1,933 men and women who were Chelsea Pensioners, and who have died whilst resident at the hospital since 29 October 2003.

About the Author

Stephen is a retired police officer having served with Essex police as a constable for thirty years between 1983 and 2013. He is married to Tanya who is also his writing partner.

This is the second book that Stephen and Tanya have co-written, their previous effort being *Women in the Great War* which was published in March 2017. Tanya has her first solo writing effort coming out in 2018, entitled, *Kent at War, 1939-45*.

Both Stephen's sons, Luke and Ross, were members of the armed forces, collectively serving five tours of Afghanistan between 2008 and 2013. Both were injured on their first tour which led to his first book, *Two Sons in a Warzone – Afghanistan: The True Story of a Father's Conflict*, which was published in October 2010.

Both of Stephen's grandfathers served during, and survived, the First World War, one with the Royal Irish Rifles, the other in the Mercantile Marine, whilst his father was a member of the Royal Army Ordnance Corps during the Second World War.

Stephen collaborated with one of his writing partners, Ken Porter, on a book published in August 2012, *German POW Camp 266 – Langdon Hills* which spent six weeks as the number one best-selling book in Waterstones, Basildon between March and April 2013. They have also collaborated on four books in the Towns and Cities in the Great War' series by Pen and Sword. Stephen has also written other titles for the same series of books as well as three crime thrillers, published between 2010 and 2012, which centre around a fictional detective named Terry Danvers.

When they are not writing, Stephen and Tanya enjoy walking their four German Shepherd dogs early each morning when most sensible people are still asleep.

Sources

Wikipedia
www.cwgc.co.uk
www.ancestry.co.uk
www.nelsonlambertblogspot.co.uk
www.british-history.ac.uk
www.billiongraves.com
www.pepysdiary.com
www.britishnewspaperarchive.co.uk
www.oglekin.org
www.hansard.millbanksystems.com
www.chelsea-pensioners.co.uk
www.britishexecutions.co.uk
A Village in Chelsea – David Ascoli. (1974)
The Royal Hospital Chelsea – Lieutenant Colonel Newnham-Davis (1912)
The Royal Chelsea Hospital (1947)

Index

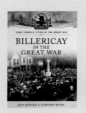
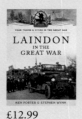
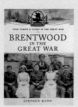
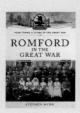
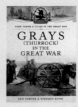
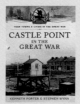
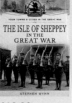
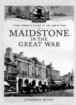
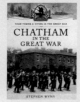

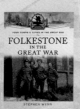
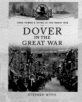
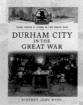
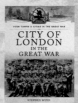
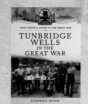
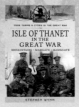
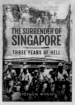
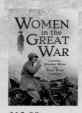
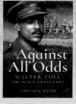